AFTER
BREAST CANCER

AFTER BREAST CANCER

A COMMON-SENSE GUIDE TO LIFE AFTER TREATMENT

Hester Hill Schnipper, LICSW, BCD

Joanie B. Hatcher Survivorship Professor
The Susan G. Komen Breast Cancer Foundation

Foreword by
Lowell E. Schnipper, M.D.

BANTAM BOOKS
New York   Toronto   London   Sydney   Auckland

AFTER BREAST CANCER: A COMMON-SENSE GUIDE TO LIFE AFTER TREATMENT
A Bantam Book / October 2003

Published by
Bantam Dell
a division of
Random House, Inc.
New York, New York

Library of Congress Cataloging in Publication Data

Schnipper, Hester Hill.
After breast cancer : a common-sense guide to life after treatment /
Hester Hill Schnipper; foreword by Lowell E. Schnipper.
p. cm.
Includes bibliographical references and index.
ISBN 0-553-38162-8
1. Breast—Cancer—Popular works.   2. Breast—Cancer—Patients—
Rehabilitation.   I. Schnipper, Lowell E.   II. Title.

RC280.B8S349 2003
616.99'44903—dc21   2003048015

Manufactured in the United States of America
Published simultaneously in Canada

10 9 8 7 6 5 4 3 2 1
RRH

For Lowell

Who shares and lives our dream

And

For Katharine and for Julia

Who will find their own

Contents

Foreword   ix

Preface   1

1   My Personal Journey   7

2   Finishing Treatment: The Very First Weeks   15

3   The Aftermath: Managing the Early Months   39

4   Physical Recovery   51

5   Medical Follow-Up   83

6   Hormonal Therapies   103

7   Complementary Therapies   118

8   Concerns of Husbands and Partners   132

9   Sexuality   146

10 Fertility and Pregnancy   166

11 Children   175

12 Parents   191

13 Friends   199

14 Professional Issues   207

15 Breast Cancer Gene and Genetic Testing   220

16 The Hard Part   236

17 Getting Support   249

18 Spirituality and Faith   263

19 Life After Breast Cancer   272

    Afterword and Resources   283

    Index   291

Foreword

I write these words as a physician who has specialized in oncology for many years and as a husband who ten years ago
found that his beloved was stricken with the disease that
had long been one of his chief professional commitments.
This experience changed me. My perceptions of caring for
women with breast cancer have been forged in the furnace
of Hester's experience. I now see every patient through the
prism of a long professional life and the anxiety of a devoted partner.

The moment a woman hears a diagnosis of breast cancer, her world is forever different. Initially stunned to the
point of numbness, she gradually finds an equilibrium that
enables her to wind her way through a complex process.
She is called upon to sift through an overwhelming amount
of information and to make difficult decisions about treatment choices so she can arrive at the options that are best
for her. While that process is all-consuming, the help of a

team of surgical and medical oncologists offers most women a structure of relationships that conveys a sense of security, if not well-being.

When the chemotherapy or radiation therapy that follows surgery is completed, however, many women experience a renewed sense of vulnerability. The awareness that there are no tests available to prove whether or not the breast cancer therapy has been fully successful provokes anxiety and often depression. The uncomfortable and image-altering effects of therapy are slow to recede, and they take their toll on the sense of womanhood, on being a partner in a relationship and a sexual being. And inevitably underlying all of this is an existential anxiety that at the least is distracting and at most can be paralyzing.

Women need to understand that these feelings are normal; they are not unique, are usually transitional, and can be dealt with. They need to know about the physical realities of their bodies now that treatments have concluded. And most importantly, they need help in integrating the cancer experience into the context of their lives in ways that enable them to grow and evolve, so that they come to see the future as an opportunity and can act on it while not denying the uncertainties that the cancer experience has introduced. They need a guide to negotiate the difficult waters of survivorship, and this is why Hester decided to write this book.

In the aftermath of breast cancer treatment, the body begins to renew itself, but the spirit takes an undulating course. While I realized this before Hester was diagnosed, that recognition was transformed by her illness. Not uncommonly, the first post-chemotherapy visit with a patient would bring me into the examination room expecting a re-lieved countenance. Not so fast! That effect is tentative if present at all, and what I more often see is someone overtly sad and scared. It's as though the "hair shirt" of chemother-apy that was just removed had been a coat of armor. How to convince her that its protection can be enduring? How to encourage engagement in life rather than retreat; how to instill confidence in the face of vulnerability? There was a time when I believed that my words alone would suffice. No longer. Greater wisdom set in after Hester's cancer. Now I sit with my patients, sometimes hand in hand, and empathize with the fear while coaxing them to point toward the future. Words are not magic, not even mine, but light at the end of the tunnel can be seen only when the eyes are open. And they *will* open, once the darkest of the shadows recede. It is then that the sense of possibilities reemerges. As a patient once told me, memorably, "To dance with death, to weep over it, to rage at it, even to laugh at it, brings a kind of resolution, an encounter with mortality that is truly a life-changing event."

Never again will life be the same—not mine, and cer-tainly not Hester's. The future is riddled with ifs, certainty an evanescent memory. But there is a new immediacy to our life: hers alone, mine alone, and ours together. The gold-and-platinum bands we had made prior to her surgery, and have worn since, have become the metaphor that binds us to each other. Officially, our wedding occurred on the first day of a New Year, and then we flew off to the Serengeti. Very often, my lighthearted but serious admoni-tion to women embarking on a course of chemotherapy is to plan a trip at the beginning and to take it when you're done. It's a restorative: a prescription marking the end of the beginning, and beginning again.

So we did that. And on a field in the Ngorongoro Crater, there was a zebra lying so still against the grass that I mistook her for dying. But moments later, as we watched, we saw her stand up—and clearly visible was a limb protruding from her bottom. Repeatedly, for three hours, she lay down on the grass, then stood, alternately resting and pushing. And then, at last, there was a foal at her side, tremulous but erect and ready to take its place in the herd. It was a sign, an unmistakable sign, that reinforced all we had come to hope for since the beginning of our journey back from despair.

There are many moments when the drama, fears, and satisfactions of the workplace reverberate at home—how could they not? But since 1993, the innocent question, "How was your day?" has a different resonance. I for one have grown in my respect and admiration for the human spirit. It emanates from those with whom I sit during the day, and from her, my soul mate—grit in the face of fear, character in the presence of the abyss, joy in the recognition of uncertainty. This is the heroism of an everyday life.

And for me, as I think of that heroism? I am reminded of Dr. Rieux in Camus' *The Plague*, at the tail end of an epidemic in a small Algerian town. Many have fallen but many remain, and they reemerge from their isolation:

And it was in the midst of shouts rolling against the terrace wall in waves that waxed in volume and duration, while cataracts of colored fire fell thicker through the darkness, that Dr. Rieux resolved to compile this chronicle so that he should not be one of those who hold their peace, but should bear witness in favor of the plague-stricken people so that some memorial of the injustice and outrage done them might endure; and to state quite simply what we learn in time of pestilence: that there are more things to admire in men (and women) than to despise—nonetheless, he knew the tale he had to tell could not be one of final victory, it could only be the record of what had had to be done, and what assuredly would have to be done again in the never ending fight against terror and its relentless onslaughts, despite their personal afflictions, by all who, while unable to be saints, but refusing to bow down to pestilence, strive their utmost to be healers.

Lowell E. Schnipper, M.D.
Evelyn and Theodore Berenson Professor of Medicine
Harvard Medical School
Chief, Division of Hematology/Oncology
Beth Israel Deaconess Medical Center

AFTER
BREAST CANCER

Preface

"Write a book about the hard part." "Why doesn't anyone tell you about what to expect?" I have been asked so often. "There is so much written for newly diagnosed women and so little for those of us who are falling apart afterward." I hear these and similar statements almost daily from women who are recovering from breast cancer.

The experience of completing active cancer treatment and beginning the rest of your life is often excruciatingly difficult. Many women are unprepared for the psychological and physical difficulties that await them in the months and years ahead. My personal experience, as well as that of the many women with whom I work, suggests that the crisis does not abate with the final chemotherapy or radiation treatment. Indeed, in many ways, the real crisis is just beginning.

In 1999, the Susan G. Komen Breast Cancer Foundation recognized the enormous challenges facing breast cancer survivors with the establishment of the Joanie B. Hatcher Survivorship Professorship. It was initially envisioned as a way to support research into quality-of-life or physical issues of survivors; then it was expanded to include the work of a clinician–survivor who spends her days in the front lines of the breast cancer fight.

When I first learned of it, I naively assumed that not just scientists but clinicians—those of us who work directly with patients—would be considered for the opening. I submitted a formal application, together with letters of support from both professional colleagues and from patients who were breast cancer survivors. It was only after I applied that I learned that the planned focus of the professorship was on scientific or medical research that involved the many issues facing breast cancer survivors. The committee had not intended to consider someone like me—a clinician–survivor who spends her days taking care of women who have breast cancer. Although I was not privy to the selection process, I can imagine that the survivors on the committee said something like: "Wait, this is important, too." And indeed, the members felt so strongly about the importance of psychosocial issues that they decided to grant two professorships: one to Dr. Patricia Ganz of UCLA, who is well known for her interest and research in survivors' issues, and one to me.

I am very grateful to the Komen Foundation for this opportunity to share what I have learned from so many. Life after breast cancer is a continuing challenge and too often a puzzle. There has been limited research or writing about the issues, both physical and emotional, faced by breast cancer survivors. Working for more than twenty years with thousands of women has enabled me to observe, learn, and teach others about the after-cancer experience. This book continues women's age-old tradition of reaching out to and helping one another. Whether or not we speak directly to one another, each of us is the repository and the conduit for all we have heard from others. Those of us who are living the experience know best what it is like and what helps us.

This book has been possible only because of the support and assistance of many people. My thanks for the solution and the time to write go to the director of my department at the Beth Israel Deaconess Medical Center, Barbara Sarnoff Lee, LICSW. My colleagues in Oncology Social Work, especially Frank McCaffrey, LICSW, cheerfully covered my practice on the days that I was working on the book. Lynn C. Franklin, the agent who took a chance on me, and Robin Michaelson, the editor who agreed to take on the book, are responsible for my work being published. I am especially grateful to Ann Harris, my editor, who cajoled, encouraged, and helped me every page of the way. This is a better book because of her work.

I am indebted to Dr. Nadine Tung for her review and comments regarding breast cancer and genetic risk. I am even more indebted to her for being my doctor. No matter what the future holds, I feel safe in her hands and her heart.

Jane Hyman was the first believer in the importance of what I have to say. Joanne Baron, Denise Bisaillon, Judi Hirshfield-Bartek, RN, and Wendy Mason of the Susan G. Komen Breast Cancer Foundation also read the manuscript and made valuable comments and suggestions.

I thank Laurie Gass, Jan Montgomery, Judith Ross, and Judith Zorfass for permission to use their poems and essay.

The women with whom I work, my sisters in this unwelcome sorority, and most especially the women who participate in my Wednesday post-treatment support group contributed their wisdom and their words.

All of the women with breast cancer whom I have known and loved over the past twenty-four years are represented in these pages. Their experiences shaped mine. I think especially of those women who have died from this disease, Betsy Lehman in particular, and I know we survivors are standing on their shoulders.

Thinking about my own life with breast cancer, I must acknowledge that my friends deserve most of the credit for my coping. In addition to Nadine Tung, M.D., I owe my life to Rosemary Duda, M.D., and Jay Harris, M.D. Dianne Holland Sullivan, RN, first and foremost my friend, later my chemotherapy nurse, and all my other colleagues in the Division of Oncology sustained me. I will be forever grateful to Vivienne and Dean Aldrich for their generosity, particularly at the time of my surgery. Stan Berman should go straight to heaven for what he did for us. Judi Bieber knows that she got me through the first horrible weeks, and Ginny Mead Hoverman never missed a chance to be my best old friend. Joan McNerney sent the totem she had carried for the ten years she had been living with cancer and a note telling me to *Pass it on in a decade*. My mother and my father, West Point to the core, taught me that "Duty, Honor, Country" can be expressed in many ways, and that grit can and must be ladylike. My brothers, Jim and Dick Lampert, have been the fans and protectors that big brothers are meant to be. My beloved daughters, Katharine and Julia, have always been at the center of my heart; how lucky I am to be related to them. One true blessing of the past decade has been gaining stepchildren; Merritt, Deborah, and Claudia enrich my world.

Most of all, I thank my husband, Dr. Lowell Schnipper, for reading every word of this manuscript, for ensuring its medical accuracy, and for challenging me always to be my best. To use his phrase, together we are cartographers of the heart. I could not have written this book or lived this life without him.

In my office, I keep a basket of rocks and shells. Each of these treasures was contributed by a woman who has had breast cancer. They were collected all over the world as women returned from their travels with a special rock to add to the basket. When I first meet with a woman who has breast cancer, I ask her to choose a rock. I suggest that she keep it with her throughout her breast cancer experience as a very special totem and a symbol of our shared good wishes. Over and over, women tell me that the rock stays with them always. In such ways do we learn the power of symbols and the power of our shared sisterhood.

Like the rocks, this book represents all that I have learned from so many wonderful women. It comes from them, through me, to you.

I

My Personal Journey

As hard as it is to remember, there was a before. I had lived for forty-four years and thought of myself as having been lucky. I had been a daughter, a sister, a wife, a mother, a lover, and a friend. I ate right, exercised, got enough sleep, and in general took good care of myself. I had been working as an oncology social worker for more than fifteen years and had recently fallen in love with a wonderful man who happened to be a medical oncologist. It usually seemed a good thing that we shared so much of our work lives and could help and understand each other. Spending our days in the midst of cancer, as we both did, we recognized and appreciated our own good health and good fortune.

I had lived through the death of my beloved father, my mother's aging and increasing needs, the loss of too many patients and friends to cancer. I had come through a divorce and was hopeful that my daughters and I were moving forward toward better times. My older daughter was clearly thriving in college, and my younger girl was a typical twelve-year-old, wondering about boys and friendships and whether I could drive her to the mall on Friday evening.

When I try to remember who I was and how my life was before breast cancer, I think especially of my work. My hospital, Beth Israel Deaconess Medical Center in Boston, has always been a well-known and respected center for breast cancer treatment. When I began to work there in 1979, it was one of only three institutions in the country where some women with certain forms of the disease were regularly offered the choice of a wide excision (lumpec-tomy) and radiation therapy rather than mastectomy. Many women came from distant cities to avail themselves of this breast-conserving option. The diagnosis and treatment of breast cancer was an institutional priority and quickly be-came my passion.

In the years since then, I have developed a wonder-ful and well-respected psychosocial support program for women who have breast cancer. With the overarching goal always empowerment and community, I have met with women and their families for counseling, facilitated count-less support groups for women in all stages of breast cancer, developed a model peer-support program called Patient to Patient, Heart to Heart, and offered many special programs. I have been active in many national breast cancer and professional organizations and have lectured widely. I have been on the faculty at the Harvard Medical School and the Boston University School of Social Work. Additionally, I have written numerous professional articles about psy-chosocial aspects of breast cancer and, following my own diagnosis, about my dual perspective and experience as patient and clinician.

Through the years, I have known and loved hundreds of women with breast cancer. I have spent thousands of hours with them and with their families as they learned to cope with their disease and its treatment. I have kept watch by too many bedsides as women died of this illness, and I have grieved later with their husbands and children. I have always had an enormous respect for the power of breast cancer and never underestimated its strength and guile.

My style with my patients had always been one of relatively few rigid boundaries and of shared human relationships, but my own diagnosis of cancer shattered any lingering walls between us and set up a new paradigm of truly working together. Whether in individual sessions in my office or in groups, we together, sharing our strength, turned to face down the tiger. We rebuilt our lives and we eventually came to appreciate the clarity that cancer brings. My own vision gradually expanded to include a life lived in parallel: therapist and patient, caregiver and care recipient. My strongest alliances shifted to stand with my patients rather than with my professional colleagues. I live a double life.

We who work for long years in oncology learn the lessons that our patients have to teach. We know that life is fragile and fleeting. We know that there is no true safety, that our insistence on healthy diets, exercise, and stress management are illusions of control. We understand that there are no real differences between our patients and us except that they have already received a diagnosis of a life-threatening illness. One of my surgeon friends tells his patients, "We are all pre-op." Unlike most people, we spend our workdays immersed in illness and death and keenly appreciate the fact that life can change or end in a moment. Denial is not an option.

There is something else. We who work long in oncology, whether we are doctors or nurses or social workers, believe at some subconscious magical level that we have struck a bargain with the gods. Of course we understand intellectually that this is not so, but in our hearts the pact has been sealed. We take on seemingly endless loads of sadness; we carry others' hope; we give and we do and we know that one person can make a difference. We spend our days trying to heal others. This is supposed to buy us, and those whom we love, protection.

For years, in both my professional and my personal lives, I had said, "*When* I get breast cancer . . ." When asked by my patients if I had been through the experience, I always answered, "Not yet." I sometimes sat with my breast cancer support groups and wondered how each of the women there had first discovered her cancer and how I would someday find my own. Why did I feel that way? My mother had breast cancer in her mid-sixties, was treated and stayed well, and no one else in my family had breast or ovarian cancer. Hardly anyone in my extended family had ever had any kind of cancer at all.

No one would have considered me to be part of a high-risk family. Being the daughter of a woman who had postmenopausal breast cancer does not appreciably increase one's risk. Why was I so certain?

During the fall of 1992 and early winter of 1993, I felt vaguely unwell. There was nothing that I could pinpoint and not even anything I could describe. There was only a certainty that something was not right. Following a number of years in a difficult marriage, a separation, and a subsequent divorce that had been very hard on me as well as on my children, I was in love. For the first time in a decade, I was truly happy and felt that my life was working out. Being superstitious enough to be concerned about bringing my good fortune to the attention of the fates, I wondered whether my diffuse malaise was a defense. Was I trying to trick the heavens into thinking I had already had my share of troubles and needed no more? Could I possibly have believed that each of us is required to contend with a set amount of pain?

Sometimes I would look in the mirror and think, *Well, I am getting older. That is why I look and feel this way.* But I knew that was not it.

I have a vivid memory of stepping out of the shower on a cold morning in January 1993 and stating: "There is something seriously wrong with me." My fiancé, a medical oncologist and professor at the Harvard Medical School, tried to tell me I was wrong. He suggested that most New Englanders feel that way during the depths of winter. He told me that I was probably not getting enough sleep and certainly was working too hard. I knew he was wrong.

A few weeks later I knew the reason for my sense of foreboding. Early in the morning, still half-asleep in bed, I stretched and my hand went straight to a lump in my left breast that had never been there before. I had been compulsive for years about breast self-examination, had yearly mammograms, and I knew the landscape of my naturally lumpy breasts. This was different. In that first instant of blinding recognition, my brain and my heart and my stomach reacted as one. I knew.

Since then, I have listened as many women have told me that they knew that something was wrong before their breast cancer was detected. They simply did not feel right. Many of us know our bodies well and our instincts are apt to be correct. One woman told me of being aware of an odd odor in the months preceding her diagnosis; it disappeared when her tumor was surgically removed. Another told a story of dreaming that she had found a lump. She awakened in a panic and touched the place on her breast where the dream lump had been. There was a real lump there and it was cancer.

I wonder now whether I always had heard these stories but dismissed them. Certainly many women describe exactly the opposite situation. They say, "I had never felt better in my life at the time that my breast cancer was found." We are all different, but I now have a deep and abiding respect for women's instincts about their bodies. When someone tells me that she is sure something is wrong, I listen carefully. Often she is right.

Having spent so many years working with women who have had breast cancer, I was well educated about the issues and the impact of the disease. I knew about treatment options, side effects, statistics, and recurrence risks. I understood that breast cancer is a family disease and that everyone in the family is affected. I knew about work-life struggles, concerns about insurability, and changes in professional roles. I knew that friendships often changed, that marriages sometimes faltered, that sexuality and sense of self were always touched. I understood that fear and sadness became permanent companions. I thought I knew all about it.

The diagnosis of breast cancer brought me to my knees.

The first, the very first lesson for me was that I knew nothing about what it was really like to have breast cancer. Working with other mothers was no preparation for having to tell my own daughters of my diagnosis. Talking with other daughters was no preparation for having to tell my own mother that her worst nightmare of seeing breast cancer extend into another generation had come true. Talking with other wives was no preparation for realizing that my own beloved might someday be with another.

Mainly, there was no way to prepare for the feelings. I was overwhelmed with terror and grief and anger. I literally did not know where to put those emotions. In the first months of working as I learned to live with my own cancer, I struggled daily with the fear. How could I sit with a woman who was dying of breast cancer, a woman who had a daughter exactly the same age as my younger girl, and help her think about how best to prepare her daughter for life without a mother? How could I comfort a woman, diagnosed and treated in tandem with me, who now had widely metastatic cancer and was facing a grim and uncertain future? How could I be helpful to anyone when my own heart was pounding and my own soul was trembling?

I raged and I wept and I recognized that I had to find a way or I could not continue. I began to look at my patients and realized that I was surrounded by lessons in how to live with fear and sadness. Each day I was amid ordinary people who were doing extraordinary things; I had only to watch them and to learn. Gradually the raw intensity subsided and a way emerged to continue with life through treatment.

As the months passed and the end of chemotherapy finally arrived, I learned the second important lesson. In retrospect, the crisis of diagnosis and the difficult months of physical treatment are almost the easy part. The real challenge comes with living with breast cancer. It is clear that the goal must be to live as though the cancer will never return. Living any other way, mired in anxiety and sadness, means that the cancer wins, whether it recurs or not.

Learning how to live "as if" is the reason for this book. It is, of course, a labor of love. I am blessed to spend my days with women who are learning with me how to live, and live well, in spite of the cloud of breast cancer. As increasing numbers of women survive and live many years after treatment, the focus of attention shifts. Everything about a woman's life is changed by the experience, and the physical and psychological difficulties can be demanding. The issues of survivorship must be appreciated for what they are: the fruits of pain and the rewards of living.

2

Finishing Treatment:
The Very First Weeks

At this point you are physically exhausted and emotionally spent. You may be bald, burned, and weigh either fifteen pounds more or ten pounds less than you did at the start. When you look in the mirror, you don't look like yourself. You most certainly do not feel like yourself. You have used all of your strength and resilience to get this far yet are now facing a long and uncertain road back to health. It is a strange disease indeed that leaves you feeling far worse at the completion of treatment than you did at the time of diagnosis!

Completing active treatment for breast cancer is often an otherworldly experience. All of a sudden, you are congratulated and abruptly thrust back into the land of the well. You, of course, are not feeling well and understand that you will remain "chemically altered" for some weeks. Even if this day, your final treatment, has been circled in red on your calendar for months, you probably approach it with some uncertainty. You may be surprised that you do not feel like celebrating. You may find that you approach the final chemotherapy infusion or radiation treatment with trepidation or even sadness. Although the months of treatment may have passed very slowly and although you may have been dreaming of this moment for a long time, you are probably not truly prepared to leave behind everything about being a patient. It is an important moment, a day to remember and to ponder, but it is not a festive occasion. During the months of treatment, many women expect to feel jubilant upon finishing. They sometimes imagine bringing a cake into the radiation department on the final day or going out to dinner with friends that night. It is certainly possible that you will feel this way, but do not be surprised if, instead of relief, you feel scared and even let down.

Consider planning and experiencing a ritual to mark this passage. Jubilation and celebration may not seem appropriate, but this is a very important time, and it will help to mark it in a meaningful way. The whole point of a ritual is to honor a major experience. Your cancer diagnosis and treatment have been one of the most significant periods of your life. It can be very helpful to honor what you have been through in a ritual or ceremony that seems fitting. This can mark an ending to the time of acute crisis and a bridge to the gradual return of the rest of your life. You may want to experience this moment alone, with your family, or with other women whom you have met while going through cancer.

There are as many possibilities of rituals as there are women looking for them. Some women find satisfaction in planting a tree or spring bulbs. One young woman invited her friends to a garden party to mark the end of her treatment. The price of admission was a perennial, and, during the party, all the gifts were planted in trust of the future. I have known others who walked on the beach and were comforted by the eternity of the ocean. One woman reenacted her favorite childhood treat by ordering and eating an entire banana split. I have known women who arranged for a mass to be said or who traveled to a special church or shrine to give thanks and pray for health. Nancy walked in the woods and picked up rocks, naming each for a fear. Giving voice to the fear, she then threw it far away. A similar gesture could be writing the name of a fear or a painful moment in the sand near the tide and then watching as the water rushes through and erases it. Karen chose this ritual and told me this story: "I first wrote *Cancer, Be Gone* in the sand and then waited for a wave. The first wave actually deposited a dead crab right on top of the word *Cancer*. How moved and relieved I was when the next wave washed both away. I knew then that Someone was paying attention."

Personally, I gathered up all the empty pill bottles that had accumulated during my months of treatment, carefully arranged them in the driveway, and then drove my car over them. It was a most satisfying farewell to the pharmaceuticals!

My own treatment included a biopsy, a wide excision (or lumpectomy) and a sampling of the axillary nodes under my arm, and chemotherapy and radiation as part of a clinical trial. The chemotherapy and radiation were given concurrently. The chemo started first and, on day 15 of Cycle I, the six weeks of radiation began. The clinical question of interest to the doctors was whether this concurrent treatment intensified the effect of the radiation and whether doses of chemotherapy drugs could be maintained or even increased in this context. For me, the appeal of the trial was that the total duration of the treatment was shorter than it would have been if each treatment had been given independently. I would have to be on treatment for "only" six months instead of almost nine. I was also delighted to receive the most aggressive treatment that was offered to me at the time.

As the months passed, I became increasingly exhausted and ill. The weeks of radiation went quickly, but my skin was quite badly burned, and I ended up coated in gooey ointments and wearing gauze pads stuffed in a most peculiar net that I pulled over my head and onto my red and oozing chest. My chemotherapy included taking one of the drugs, Cytoxan, in pill form, and I was stunned by the power of anticipatory nausea. By the fourth or fifth month, simply looking at the pill bottle or holding the tablets in my hand stimulated dry heaves. Hypnosis helped some with the nausea, but the power of the mind was demonstrated by an incident toward the end of my treatment. Standing in front of the washing machine, I opened a new box of detergent. It was white with blue speckles, exactly the same coloration as the Cytoxan pills. I promptly threw up into the washing machine!

Throughout, I worked hard to sustain the fantasy that I was in control and that life was more or less normal. That meant that I went to work every day, drove my daughter and her friends to the mall, went out on weekends, and occasionally cooked dinner.

In retrospect, I did myself a major disservice by not reducing my obligations, slowing down a little, and learning to be gentle with myself. The cost of my unrelenting standards was physical and emotional depletion. I crawled to the finish and then could not understand why I felt so badly. It was almost impossible to remind myself what I had told so many other women who reported a similar sense of despair at the end of their active treatment.

My twelfth and final chemotherapy infusion took place, as usual, in the late afternoon. Continuing my stubborn routine of trying to maintain business as usual, I then went to an American Cancer Society Board of Trustees meeting. I had long been a board member and especially wanted to go that day because I was scheduled to give a short report. I cannot recall what I spoke about; I do remember that I still had the bandage on my hand where the IV had been only a few hours earlier. I vividly remember feeling exhausted, somewhat queasy, exhilarated, and terrified all at once. I also remember that I cried in the car all the way home. This is definitely not the recommended way to mark your last treatment!

Sometimes it becomes obvious only later that these very early days were mismanaged. Sara, a fifty-four-year-old college professor, came to talk with me several months after completing her chemotherapy and radiation treatments. She described herself as feeling increasingly worse psychologically as she became stronger physically and identified these feelings as coinciding with the end of her treatment. Throughout, she had continued to work and made very few changes in her daily routine. It was clearly a point of pride that "cancer did not rule my life." But now that she "should" be feeling better, she found instead that she was tearful, fragile, and furious at many people who loved her. Her most intense anger, to her horror, was directed at her husband, who had been "unbelievably supportive" through-out her medical ordeal. As we talked about him and about their obviously positive relationship, she described his ac-companying her to all of her appointments, crying with her, holding her, and helping her feel that she was not going through cancer alone. It was only as we thought together about his reactions at the completion of her treatment that she began to understand the roots of her anger. The evening of her final radiation therapy, he surprised her with reser-vations to a favorite and special restaurant and insisted that they go out together "to celebrate." She had been too ex-hausted and upset to decline this invitation at the time, but the evening did not go well, and she had continued semi-consciously to resent his perception of this as a "celebra-tion." She realized that, ever since that day, he had acted as though she had "beaten the cancer and should be happy about that." She, of course, was living instead with constant foreboding, anxiety, and real grief. She found his complete misunderstanding of her feelings a total loss of empathy, an emotional abandonment at a time when she needed him most. As she came to understand this dynamic and then to speak with her husband about her feelings, her overall emo-tional state began to improve.

Speaking to me a few months after completing her treatment, Julia described it this way: "Here's how I am: fu-rious, exhausted, overwhelmed, scared, sad, and fat." Like Julia, you are likely to experience some or most of those feelings in the months to come. Their intensity makes you feel out of control. The roller coaster of your moods and your feelings is frightening as you wonder when, if ever, you will feel more settled. Over and over in this book, I will reassure you that all of these feelings are normal and that over time you will gradually feel better.

Think back to the first days after you learned that you had breast cancer. It probably felt then as though your world had turned upside down and inside out. Terror and grief overwhelmed you. The hours seemed endless and you wondered how you would make it through the first day, the first week, the months of treatment stretching ahead of you. There was no time then to contemplate the years after that. The rest of the world, all the things that normally interested and occupied your time, faded into unimportance. All you could think about was your diagnosis and the overpowering feelings that controlled you. It seemed as if never again would you pass an hour, let alone a whole day, without thinking of your cancer. It was your last thought at night and your first thought in the morning. It was also likely your only thought during wakeful hours in the middle of the night.

You may have had trouble sleeping, either unable to get to sleep at night or awakening in the dark early morning to worry. Some women remember spending these sleepless hours planning who might care for their children after their death or what music they wanted at their funeral. One woman said she spent the hours between 2:00 and 4:00 A.M. regularly evaluating the women she knew as the potential next wife for her husband. You may have lost your appetite or, perhaps, could not stop eating. You may have told everyone you met about your cancer diagnosis or may have found it difficult to even tell your family and close friends. Medical information and choices, cancer vocabulary, frightening statistics, and the need to make treatment decisions were probably overwhelming you. You may have received far too much reading material and advice from friends or you may have chosen to read nothing other than what your doctors gave you. You must have cried a lot and wondered whether, ever again, you would laugh and feel like yourself. Your life was out of control.

We know from psychological-crisis theory that an acute crisis cannot last more than a few weeks. No matter what the stresses, no matter what the situation, human beings are amazingly resilient and adaptable and in time begin to find a way to live with their new life circumstances. Situations and problems that would previously have seemed impossible to tolerate begin to seem almost normal. People somehow find the psychological and practical resources to keep on living and to develop new routines and perspectives that enable them to cope. A friend whose daughter was being treated for leukemia said to me, "You get used to anything." Looking back, you can see this was true for you, too.

If you were lucky in those early weeks of many medical appointments, difficult decisions, and powerful feelings, someone assured you that you would feel better once a little time had passed and you had begun your treatments. It is unlikely that you believed the messenger at the time, but you discovered that it was true. As hard as it is for a newly diagnosed woman to believe, life does start to feel better relatively quickly. You chose your doctors, decided about your surgery and other treatments, and slowly a routine evolved that gave you a little more control. You learned what to anticipate after a chemotherapy treatment, which antinausea drugs worked best for you. If you lost your hair, you found a wig or hats or scarves and the courage to go out in public. After a while, you probably stopped covering your head at home and discovered, to your astonishment, that your kids rather liked your bald head.

Carol, a sixty-year-old psychologist, spoke to me on the morning of the day after her last radiation-therapy treatment. She began by describing the feeling of having no place special to go, no particular plan for the day. After weeks of getting up early for an 8:00 A.M. radiation appointment, she suddenly had a free morning. She said, "Everyone is congratulating me on getting through it and putting it behind me, and I feel that I have only just begun. My daughter asked whether I felt 'relieved,' and I wondered, 'Relieved about what?' She assumes that since all the treatments are over, I must be cured. And I wonder whether the surgery got all the cancer out and whether, because of the two positive lymph nodes, there is still some cancer floating around in my body. My son and his fiancée congratulated me, and, although I feel good about having tolerated everything quite well, I am not at all sure that I succeeded at anything! (Isn't that usually when we get congratulated?) When I obsess with my husband about whether the cancer is going to return, he, in his quiet way, tells me that I am probably fine.

"If I could be certain that the cancer were gone, then I guess I could learn to look at this as an isolated period in my life. But I don't think that is possible. Even if some people can do this, having cancer is a life-changing experience—so how can it ever be viewed as 'isolated' from the rest of one's life?"

The months of treatment were difficult. Carol eloquently described some of the reasons why the months following treatment are difficult, too. While you were dealing with chemotherapy or radiation or recovering from surgery, you learned to listen to your body. The physical demands were primary. Living daily with fatigue or nausea or pain forced you to pay close attention to the structure of your days and to plan how to best use your physical energy and resources. You prioritized your tasks; you may have changed your work schedule. You accepted offers of help and you even learned how to ask for assistance. You managed! As your treatment ends and you no longer need to contend with the intense physical symptoms, multiple medical appointments, and a calendar filled with cancer, you will find that all the rest of your life demands your attention. You will probably also find that you will only *very* slowly begin to know how to think about your life in all of its angst and glory.

Many women find that, during the months of active treatment, they are so consumed by the physical needs and demands that they have little energy for the psychological issues that breast cancer brings. For years I have facilitated a support group for women undergoing adjuvant chemotherapy: chemotherapy that is given in the context of no known remaining cancer but as an insurance policy to protect against any cancer cells that might be somewhere in the body. The group is a place for them to feel understood and to gather helpful information regarding their treatments and day-to-day coping. The women in this group usually feel that they could not have managed without it or without the warm companionship of the others there.

Some years ago, four women who had been coming to this treatment support group asked if they could meet with me at a different time. They said they felt they needed to move on, that the concerns expressed by newly diagnosed women who were embarking on chemotherapy were different from the ones they were experiencing now. Somewhat to their surprise, they were having a harder time emotionally than they had during their treatments. What about a post-treatment support group?

So I began a new after-treatment support group, and it quickly became so crowded that we divided into two groups. These two groups, with a changing population, have continued ever since, and I am always profoundly moved by what I hear in those sessions. Of course, to be fully honest, the concerns of women who are trying to figure out how to live their lives after breast cancer are the same concerns with which I struggle. My identification with these women and these groups is strong. I continue to be reminded weekly that most women begin to deal with the psychological impact of their disease only after the months of active treatment. Over and over, they tell me that this transition is the hardest part and that there are few signposts or guides to point the way.

One of my patients described the time of diagnosis as feeling like "the perfect storm," full of panic and chaos and terror. The months of treatment that follow, she said, are like riding a barge down a canal: slow but steady, guided from the shores, the route clear and laid out in front of you.

But finishing treatment is like coming out the other end of the canal into the open sea. The weather may be placid or stormy, the forecasts are unreliable, and you are on your own to navigate.

But navigate you must. One of my patients described a dream that powerfully expressed her feelings as she finished treatment. In her dream, she was in a room with a number of friends who wanted to talk with her about cancer. She kept trying to change the subject and finally realized that she would have to leave. As she turned to run, she discovered that she was wearing sneakers and that their shoelaces were tied together. She was trapped. Try as you might, you cannot leave your cancer experience behind. Running won't help!

At the time of initial diagnosis, you may have felt overwhelmed by information and advice. There are many excellent books written to help with that difficult period. There is much less that addresses what comes afterward. You may be feeling quite alone.

This book is about your new life. You will never be the same woman you were before you had cancer. Your life will never be the same. Longing for what was will not return it to you. Instead, you slowly find your way to something different. Christine described it this way: "When I think of myself and how it is now, I would say *emerging spirit* or something like that. My life after breast cancer is an ongoing journey of discovery about who I am now and who I will become. I think that will never end, because everything that impacts me is viewed with renewed insight. The person I am now continues to evolve but will eternally, silently be guided by my experience with breast cancer."

Trying to find words to describe this new life can be difficult. Ann called it "the pervasive poignancy of life after breast cancer." Kay discovered that three-letter acronyms are often used in computer chat rooms and began to call her situation "life abc" or "life after breast cancer." Pat described "a new awareness of life that translates to recognizing what is important to me, who is important to me, and what I want to do with my life since I know that the disease may come back and end my life."

Any major life experience changes us, and breast cancer has almost certainly changed you physically, emotionally, and spiritually. You do not look quite the same; even after your hair is back, you will have a few scars you did not have before this all began. What was once normal and routine becomes what we hope for but cannot necessarily count on. You will measure "normal" differently; Denise calls it "normal plus." You have learned a great deal about your capacity for strength, for courage, for empathy, and for love. You are certain to make some decisions and life choices differently than you would have had the cancer not happened. Years ago I worked with a psychiatrist who liked to say, "Adults grow only on the rack." He meant that all of us are somewhat fixed in our ways and resistant, to a greater or lesser degree, to change. We grow through pain, when we are forced to do so. You have known pain and you have grown. Your new you is a self that has expanded to hold these experiences. It is a self that will become comfortable, familiar, and very beloved over time.

But right now that kind of strength, that recovered and sturdy you, lies in the future. Instead of feeling that they have resumed their normal life a few months after finishing treatment, many women find that they are more frightened, sad, and emotionally out of balance than ever. Mary Ellen described it this way: "So this must be phase three. I am having realizations about my family, my friends, myself. I guess this cancer thing really brings to light a lot of stuff you aren't prepared for in addition to the basic fear of dying. There are so many phases! First, the diagnosis and treatment. Second, the after-treatment blues and adjustment, and now, third, the 'realizations.' What is this phase called? My husband calls it 'phase three of lumpy gravy.' It's a line from an old rock song, but neither of us can remember which one."

Many of us even have difficulty with the language of these days. What is the right word to use? Do you *have* cancer? Is *had* the better term? Are you a *survivor*, or does that term make you superstitious and nervous? As silly as this may seem, the words are important. They are how you present and define yourself to the world. You will eventually find the language that feels best for you; it may evolve and change over time. Personally, I am very uncomfortable with the *survivor* word. Generally, I say something like, "I was treated for breast cancer in 1993." That phrase sidesteps the choice of the verb tense and feels safer to me.

As much as you hated radiation and chemotherapy, it brought with it a sense of security. How could any cancer possibly grow in your body while those powerful chemicals were flowing through you? How could any cells left in your breast possibly survive those radiation rays? But, with active treatment now completed, most women become preoccupied and apprehensive about their health. What if there is a single cancer cell lurking somewhere? Did the chemotherapy work? How does anyone know if it worked? How will my doctors follow me and how will they know if the cancer comes back?

Since every woman's cancer and every woman's treatment is uniquely her own, no woman's recovery will exactly parallel any other's. The particular combination of surgery, radiation, chemotherapy, or hormonal therapy that you had will to some extent influence the course of your recovery.

Women who do not receive chemotherapy but whose treatment involves surgery with or without radiation and hormonal therapy—usually tamoxifen—face a slightly different adjustment. Although they have been spared the rigors of chemotherapy, they have also had less time and less public recognition of what they were going through. No one enjoys being bald and feeling sick, but that reality does mean that people around you see what you are experiencing. Since chemotherapy is usually given over a period of three to six months, you also have time to adapt to being a breast cancer patient and to process the strong feelings that always accompany the diagnosis.

But women who do not have chemotherapy sometimes find that their family and friends have relatively little understanding of what they have experienced. Throughout the course of their treatment, any physical side effects or scars are hidden from the world. Skin burns from radiation and scars from surgery, even a mastectomy, are invisible. And since most women try hard to sustain their usual responsibilities and routines, it is easy for others to minimize the impact of the experience.

Moreover, women in this situation may feel that they

have no right to complain because they have not had to endure the rigors of chemotherapy. Sitting in a support group or in a waiting room with others who have, they may feel that they do not quite belong and that their "luck" isolates them from other breast cancer patients. There can be a very unfortunate sense of a breast cancer hierarchy that works in both directions. On the one hand, it is better to have had an early-stage or even a preinvasive (DCIS or LCIS) cancer. On the other, having a high-risk breast cancer with multiple positive lymph nodes and heavy-duty treatment can "trump" everyone else's experience. It is important to remember that the feelings about having breast cancer are completely independent from the treatment. Women who have had a tiny tumor excised and need only radiation can have the same feelings as women with high-risk breast cancer who require multiple therapies including a stem-cell transplant. Any kind of breast cancer and any kind of treatment are bad enough!

Women who have had more extensive treatment may find it easier to express their difficulties. Sandy, a thirty-seven-year-old social worker, said: "It has been four months since I ended my radiation therapy. For me, finishing treatment brought up so many issues. I am trying to figure out where and how I now fit into the world. I had been actively a cancer patient for ten months, and now I don't have a doctor's appointment for four months. It is a confusing time.

"My partner wants me to increase my IRA savings. Although I hope and expect to live to retirement age, I told her I could not do it this year but would next. I feel I just have to do whatever I want this year and will be more responsible next year. My expectation is that this will get eas-

ier with time, although there will always be worry and uncertainty. Learning to live with that, while not limiting my
living to the present, is my goal."

With treatment completed, many women also feel
some sense of abandonment by their health-care providers.
Frequent visits with doctors, nurses, and radiation techs
were reassuring. There was always someone available to answer a question or to reassure a fear. If your treatments
were physically demanding, and especially if you changed
your normal work or social routines, those medical con-
tacts may have become the most important relationships in
your life for those months. What now?

You are also discovering that the return to robust physical health is slow. Many women expect to feel well as soon
as treatment is over. Their friends and family also expect
them to be back to normal now and to pick up whatever
tasks or responsibilities they have surrendered during treatment. If you lost your hair, you are extremely impatient for
it to grow back to its normal length. But hair growth can
seem excruciatingly slow, and the new hair may well be different. In addition to the common post-chemotherapy curls
(which may disappear after a few months), many women
find that their hair has more gray in it or is even a different
color than they remember.

It is likely that you were so focused on getting through
your medical treatments and so busy with life as a cancer
patient that you did not really deal with the psychological
and life issues that are confronting you now. It is completely
normal and appropriate to feel depressed, anxious, and
generally out of sync with your friends and family. Their
concerns may well seem trivial to you, and it can be hard to

be sympathetic to their problems when you are worrying about your survival. Jan, only a few weeks out of the hospital following a bone-marrow transplant for her high-risk breast cancer, rode with a friend to pick up the friend's new car. All the way to the dealership, the friend complained about the need to purchase a family sedan; she actually said that she was "grieving" her inability to buy the SUV she really wanted. Jan wanted to throttle her!

You have been forever changed by your diagnosis and experience. You will never get your old life back. You will, however, build a life that may someday be even better than your old one. You *will* feel like yourself again; one morning you will awaken and think: *I remember feeling this way. This is me.* You will find laughter and pleasure and joy. Many of us actually come to believe that our lives are even fuller and more satisfying because of our cancer. This is not something that a newly diagnosed woman could ever believe. You may indeed gradually find that it is true for you.

Victoria, a forty-five-year-old mother and personal trainer, advises: "Give yourself some time. The first six months to a year after my treatment ended, I had days that were very difficult and panicky. I wondered what you are wondering: Will I be here to see my kids graduate from high school or college, will I be at their weddings? I felt very unsure and I needed to talk a lot about my experience. I know I drove a lot of my friends crazy, because I had something of a one-track mind. And some days I felt overwhelmed with sadness, and on others I felt on top of the world. It was a roller-coaster ride.

"The nice thing is that you *do* come to a better, less scary place, emotionally and physically, as time goes on.

This is a journey, and you need to take it. Everyone's path is a little different. Healing does happen—just not instantly."

Breast cancer is a wake-up call. It is the special-delivery letter that says, *You, too, are mortal. You will die someday.* All of us fervently hope that we will be lucky and will live to a ripe and healthy old age, but knowing that we may not be so fortunate gives us a chance to examine our lives. I believe that an examined life is the only life worth living, and I believe that the misfortune of breast cancer gives us the opportunity to create the life we really want.

If this does not do it, what will? If breast cancer does not shake you to your core and then toss you back into the middle of life, what could?

Judith Zorfass, an education consultant and author, wrote an essay called "My Balancing Act." Her work was included in a book of writings by cancer patients and survivors that we publish each year as part of our Celebration of Life / National Cancer Survivors' Day. Because I think she describes so well the challenge of finding a new normal, or learning to balance in a new world, I asked her permission to include it here. The search for the balance that she describes is not one that you can complete in the first days or weeks after your treatment ends. Understand that this will be a process and that the process itself will be as valuable as the goal.

My Balancing Act

Picture a large ball. A long plank of wood lies across the top of the ball. I'm standing on top trying to keep my balance. Even with my arms outstretched and my feet planted about six inches apart, I teeter-totter, teeter-totter back and forth—leaning first slightly to the left and then to the right. What I'm trying to keep in balance is forgetting and remembering, hope and despair, work and play.

Teeter-Totter. Forgetting and Remembering. Sometimes I forget within minutes of my annual mammogram that I was diagnosed with cancer. Celebrating a holiday with family, brainstorming with colleagues, dining out with my husband and friends, or becoming engrossed in a juicy novel can, for just a nanosecond, obliterate the truth from my mind. Oh, how I would love to linger in that blissful forgetfulness. But the reality of my diagnosis creeps back into my consciousness. I'm flooded with vivid images of recent surgeries, doctors' appointments, procedures, and treatments. To once again regain my balance, I force myself to close the covers of that unwanted, imaginary photo album.

Teeter-Totter. Hope and Despair. To tilt toward hope, I give myself one of those "think positive" pep talks. I repeat over and over, almost like a mantra: "Your cancer was detected early. You've received powerful therapies. You're helping yourself by eating right and exercising daily." Sometimes it works. But sometimes even these compelling words fail to ward off despair. Gnawing apprehension throws me off balance. So that's when I use one of my lifelines to prevent myself from totally succumbing to abject fear. I call upon the wisdom of my daughter, who advises, "Why waste a good day worrying about a possible bad day in the future?" Agreeing that I will not allow cancer to rob me of today, I regain my balance.

TEETER-TOTTER. WORK AND PLAY. Maintaining the balance between work and play should be the easiest to accomplish because there is finally something that is under my control. Finding passion and identity in my work, I'm your stereotypic workaholic. Traditionally, the ratio of work to play in my life's equation has been $8X + 3Y = $ Life, with X being work and Y being play. But then I ask myself the hard question: "Is this really the right equation?" Why multiply the work variable to the point of feeling overwhelmed and overtaxed? I have the power to change the equation to $3X + 8Y = $ Life. Then Y represents playing with our three gorgeous grandbabies, spending time with their mothers, our two wonderful daughters, walking on the beach holding my husband's hand, schmoozing with friends, and hunting for bargains with my sister. In my new math, reducing the work and increasing the play still results in a balanced equation.

Teeter-totter. Teeter-totter. Trying to keep my arms out straight. Teeter-totter. Teeter-totter. Trying not to lean too far one way or another. Teeter-totter. Teeter-totter. How long can I keep up my balancing act? As long as I am blessed to be here. That's what survivors do.

Creating your own new life means finding a balance in all parts of it. There will be days when you fall. There will be many days when you feel shaky. But you can be certain that, over time, there will be more and more days when you stand steady. Many women feel that breast cancer has given them a second chance. Grab it and hold on for dear life.

Here are some thoughts or actions to consider upon finishing treatment:

- You probably do not feel like celebrating at this moment (if you do, you certainly should do so!), but do think about ways to mark this important time in your life.
- Consider a ritual, either by yourself or with others, to respect your courage and your accomplishment. You have done something very, very hard.
- Remember that the effects of surgery, radiation, and chemotherapy are long-lasting. This can be reassuring.
- If you are taking tamoxifen or another hormonal therapy, remember that it, too, has powerful and long-lasting effects. You are still on anticancer therapy.
- Make your first follow-up appointment as early as your doctor recommends. You will be glad of the contact and the reassurance.
- Remind yourself that finishing treatment is very difficult and that you are entitled to some self-indulgence.
- Find and practice small ways to be nice to yourself. Keep fresh flowers in your house. Subscribe to several light magazines. Try a massage.
- In the early weeks, as your hair is slowly growing in and your complexion is gradually returning to your normal healthy skin tones, you will still need to use more makeup than you might in your ordinary routine. Hopefully, you discovered many of these tips while you were on chemotherapy. However, in case you didn't, here are some ideas that will take only a few minutes each morning. These tips were given to me by one of my patients, a former Miss Massachusetts:

1. Start with a good concealer to match your skin. In particular, use the concealer under your eyes and on any dark pigmented spots that developed during treatment.
2. A crème-to-powder base in a compact works well; it is fast and allows better control.
3. If your complexion became sallow during treatment, avoid yellow-based foundations. Go a bit pinker or use a translucent pink cheek color instead of a standard foundation.
4. Cheek color: Choose pinks over peaches or ambers if sallow skin is still a problem. If your face is fuller because of medications or weight gain, try putting blush high on the cheekbone and experiment with a darker color below.
5. Choose a lipstick from the same color family as your blush.
6. While your eyebrows are still patchy, fill them in with a pencil or brow kit. Look for a brow kit that is a pressed powder with a brush.
7. Choose a good quality (no creasing) eye shadow in a very light color as a base. If you are fair, look for colors with *sand* or *ivory* in their names. If your complexion is darker, look for *amber* or *tan*. Put this light color all over your eyelid to brighten your entire eye. If you want, you can use a darker color in the outer third of the eyelid, blending it toward the center.
8. If your eyelashes are sparse, experiment with liquid eyeliner to fill in the gaps. Do not use eyeliner under your eye unless you are well under thirty; it will "close" the eye and make you look very tired.

- Try to find and talk with a few other women who have gone through breast cancer ahead of you. They will help normalize what you are feeling and reassure you, in a believable way, that you will feel better.

- Think about easy ways to thank some of the people who have helped you through these months. Starting to give back to others will feel good.
- Learn to live your life as an exultation, not an explanation. It will take time, but the rewards will be infinite!

3

The Aftermath:
Managing the Early Months

In these first weeks and months when you are still psychologically and physically balanced somewhere between health and illness, it is all too easy to be overwhelmed. When you are barely starting to believe that there is a life ahead waiting for you, you have a unique opportunity to set priorities and establish new patterns. This is a time when you are slowly taking back your responsibilities and usual schedule. Do not do so on automatic pilot! Stop and think about what you choose and why you are choosing it. Remember what you have learned about your priorities and apply that now to building your life. Once more time has passed and you are again busy with your routine, it will be more difficult to remember what these months have taught you.

What can you expect in this period? First and foremost, you cannot expect to feel like your old self! Remember that it has taken many weeks or months just to get to this point. The basic rule of thumb is that it will take the same length of time to regain your usual sense of well-being as was the total duration of your treatment. Count the weeks from the day of your diagnosis until the day of your final treatment. That is how long it is likely to take to really feel well. This rule holds whether you had "only" surgery and radiation or whether you had many months of intensive chemotherapy. Obviously the curve is in the direction of better health and more energy, but it is not a steady course, and ahead lie many days of fatigue, worry, and frustration with the slow pace of your recovery.

The importance of this timetable cannot be overemphasized. You cannot push yourself to a full recovery any more quickly, and trying to speed it up will only result in exhaustion and stress. You may have to write this rule on an index card and tape it to your mirror: *I cannot expect to feel fully myself until March.* It is critical that you do not lose sight of the pace and rhythm of the recovery process. Cherish the days that you do feel energetic and cheerful, but do not be discouraged or self-critical on the ones when you find yourself tired and depressed.

There will be mornings when you awaken with the stunning thought: *Oh, my God, I have had cancer!* There will be moments when you experience a sudden jolt of fear. There will be moments of impatience with your family and friends. There will be moments when, for no obvious reason, you find yourself in tears. There will be times when, like Joyce, you feel, *Now it is just me and my odds.*

Finding the right balance and giving yourself permission to do this is essential in your daily life and routines. Judith, a thirty-five-year-old writer, said: "My work this summer has gone well. I did everything that I set out to do but did not go overboard. Instead of counting half of an eight-hour day as six hours (as I did in past summers), I actually forced myself to stop working after four hours." She found, as we all do, that it is actually possible to do less without the world collapsing!

Sara methodically did this. She said, "Like probably everyone who has had cancer, I have spent a fair amount of time thinking about my life and how I am living it. I finally decided that if I die too soon, I would have the following regrets:

- I don't see my friends enough.
- I continue to not exercise and not be in better physical shape.
- I don't do anything with my art.
- I've never been to France or Italy.

"I need to do something about all of those things now, because I don't plan on departing from this planet, whenever that is, with this sack of regrets. That's for sure."

With these clear goals and dreams in mind, Sara set out to change her life. She was able to negotiate a new work schedule, working forty hours in four long days. The new day of freedom that she gained was devoted to painting. She made sure that she found time to see her friends and to walk each day. Best of all, she and her husband went to France and Italy for three weeks the following summer. The trip was a financial stretch for them, but she decided that since living to an old age and then spending her retirement money was not a certainty, living well now was a priority.

Your family and friends are working from a different

mental calendar. You may quickly be asked, "When can you start working full time again?" or "Can you chair this school committee now?" or "Can't you take back your regular three mornings of driving the car pool?" I talked about these very probabilities at a session with Louise, an artist who had just completed three months of chemotherapy followed by six weeks of radiation. Although she assured me her friends would be more understanding and not assume she was ready to step right back into her old life, I insisted that she be prepared with strategies should she be wrong. When we met the next week, she told me that exactly what we discussed had indeed happened. In the intervening days, several friends had called her wanting to know whether she could chair an upcoming art show, substitute for a teacher who was unexpectedly absent, and take a friend's daughter for the weekend while her parents went away. Fortunately, she was prepared for these requests, and she used the scripts that we had talked about. But it was still hard to say no, and she was feeling both angry and guilty.

When the intense months of treatment are finished, you may also discover that you are surrounded by a myriad of life problems, large or small, that you either ignored or were unaware of while you focused on your illness. You are likely to feel even more out of control as you take stock of what lies around you. The medical bills may be piled up on your desk while normal household tasks or repairs may have been delayed for many months. The more that you see undone or poorly done, the worse you may feel. You need to remind yourself, and perhaps those around you, that your time and attention and energy have been necessarily and appropriately focused on your health over these past months. Anything that did not directly affect your treatment was unimportant. There is time now and there will be time in the future to catch up, to make repairs or amends, and to shape your life again. Jane later laughed about looking around her house in July and noticing that boots and snow shovels were still in the entryway. It can be overwhelming to feel so behind in the management of your life, so, again, you must remind yourself to go slowly and to lower your expectations.

Let me repeat that it is vital that you give yourself time and space and permission to go slowly as you move through this transition back toward your life. Remember that the people who love you want to believe that your breast cancer is over and done with, cured. It is too frightening and painful for them to think about the fact that you are still living with breast cancer and that you will never receive a promise that you have been cured. Many other illnesses and health problems are truly over when they are over, and some people don't understand that breast cancer does not work that way. Joan told me of a major fight with her husband three months after the end of her treatment. They were shopping for a wedding gift for a nephew and also bought a set of kitchen utensils for themselves. When they left the shop, Joan burst into tears. "I can't help wondering if I will even live to use that slotted spoon," she said. Her husband, frustrated and angry, kept repeating, "Stop worrying. I know you are fine." These comments, of course, served only to isolate her with her fear.

Difficult though this is to accept, the truth is that your family and friends are eager to be relieved of their worry about you and to return to their own busy lives. The result is that most women find that the strong support they receive at the time of their diagnosis begins to fade as treatment goes on and may be much diminished by the time it is completed. It is unfortunate but true that your diagnosis may soon become old news to even those close to you.

Other serious concerns, which will be discussed more fully in later chapters, may include noticing real changes or rifts in long-standing relationships. The chances are good that some of your friends were not as present for you as you would have hoped they would be. Now is the time to think about whether you want to talk with them about your hurt and disappointment, how you want to deal with the anger you are feeling, and even whether you want to expend the energy to try to repair those friendships. Family members, too, may not have behaved as you wished they would. You learned that a real crisis does not necessarily mend long-standing family conflicts or issues. Linda described never feeling close to her older brother and always wishing that they could find a way to be a more important part of each other's lives. When her breast cancer was diagnosed, he called regularly and even came to visit right after her surgery. However, as the months passed, he stopped reaching out to her so often, and by the time her treatment ended, their old patterns of rare communication had been reestablished.

For all of these reasons, it has been my experience that many women call me for the first time after completing their treatment. Although they may have been aware that psychological-support services were available to them at any point following their diagnosis, it is only now that the emotional issues seem impossible to manage alone. Kathleen, a forty-year-old nurse and mother of two, began to work with me six weeks following her final chemotherapy. A very competent and energetic woman, she was dismayed to find herself feeling vulnerable, frightened, and often fatigued. Beyond worries about numerous family, professional, and financial issues was her unsettling sense that "something is just wrong with me." Besides some practical advice on coping with her problems, the most helpful part of our work together, I believe, was the reassurance that all of her feelings were normal and that she would gradually come to feel more like herself.

Most women come in for a few therapy sessions and then begin to feel better. Like Kathleen, they need acknowledgment of their experience, normalization of their feelings, and a chance to express their fear and sadness to a neutral and supportive person. Calling a therapist is never a sign of weakness. To the contrary, it is often the smartest and strongest thing you can do for yourself. Why suffer needlessly when help is at hand?

Occasionally, women have a particularly difficult time psychologically and do not naturally and gradually regain their emotional equilibrium. While their feelings may seem to be more intense versions of what others experience, on occasion their symptoms seem to fit a syndrome called post-traumatic stress disorder, or PTSD. This is a not-uncommon human reaction to a terrible life experience and can affect survivors of any major crisis or disaster. Symptoms include difficulty sleeping, mood swings, angry outbursts, and flashbacks or intense preoccupation with the crisis. Although more commonly associated with survivors of an accident, wartime battle, or a natural disaster such as an earthquake or fire, my experience is that following breast cancer some women also have feelings and behaviors that fit this model.

Women with breast cancer who have previously experienced trauma in their lives are especially vulnerable to full-blown PTSD. If you have been a victim of childhood sexual abuse or rape or another violent crime or natural calamity, be aware that this is likely to be a particularly difficult time for you. Even if you feel that you are managing well, it would be advisable to make a connection with a therapist, meet once or twice to establish a relationship, and thus know that you have someone available to help you if the feelings become acute.

A woman need not have PTSD, however, to become depressed or anxious. Again, these are frequent reactions to this crisis. There was an old advertisement that ended with the line, *You can pay me now or you can pay me later*. I think that this fits the experience of going through breast cancer. Sooner or later, you have to deal with the emotional trauma. Some women fall apart at diagnosis, others at some point during their treatment. I believe, however, that for the majority of women, the most difficult time comes at the end of treatment.

How can you tell if your psychological recovery is more than "normally" difficult and whether you need help from a therapist as you move toward recovery? By reading this book you are, of course, learning more about normal reactions following cancer and can begin to compare your feelings with those described here. If you find that you are having difficulty sleeping, that your appetite has changed in either direction and you are gaining or losing weight, that you have lost interest in your usual activities and friends, that you have trouble concentrating, and that you are frequently tearful or angry, and if these feelings persist for several months following treatment, you should consider talking with a therapist. As a general rule, if you wonder if this would be helpful, it will be. Chapter 17, "Getting Support," discusses more fully finding and working with the right therapist. As is always true, it is important to work with a therapist who is knowledgeable and competent *and* who is someone you like. The human chemistry is vital.

A few weeks after my own final chemotherapy treatment, I traveled with my fiancé and his daughter to his father's eightieth birthday party. In retrospect, I should have paid attention to my vague sense that this was a mistake and that I was not strong enough to take on this potentially emotion-filled event. The situation was even more complicated because his twenty-one-year-old daughter and I were just getting to know each other and were carefully navigating the potential land mines of an upcoming second marriage. The first problem developed almost immediately. Trying to be polite, I suggested that she ride in the front seat with her father. I realized later that I did not expect her to actually do this and I certainly did not realize that I would be furious. Huddled in the backseat, tired, vulnerable, and thin-skinned, I was lost in miserable fantasies of recurrent cancer and premature death.

By the time we stopped at the hotel to change our clothes and then go on to the party, I was barely in control of my strong feelings. Again, I should have paid attention to how close to collapse I was; I should have stayed behind in the hotel to recover. Instead, trying as always to do what was expected of me, I went on with them to the party. It was a lovely and festive dinner in a restaurant in a parklike setting, but midway through the meal, I bolted from the room and started to run down a nearby path. Stumbling in high heels and blinded by tears, I wailed. Never since I had learned of my breast cancer had I been so overwhelmed by emotion. Grief and fear and fury combined to set me sobbing, as I asked myself over and over how this had happened, how I had gotten through the previous six months, and how I could bear to be at an eightieth birthday party when I was not sure that I was going to live to be forty-five.

I rarely tell anyone about this horrible day and have hesitated to write about it now. However, I know that it is important to reassure you that the overpowering feelings you may be experiencing now are normal. You are not crazy. You have been through terrible times, probably holding yourself together by force of will and working hard to keep your life as stable as possible. There is bound to be an impact by now. Once the acute crisis of your diagnosis and treatment is over, you lower your psychological defenses, and it is when you let down the barriers that such feelings crash down on you.

"It's as though my life is a city that has been destroyed in a war," said Jenna, an artist who had lived through a mastectomy and six months of intensive chemotherapy. "All of the landmarks are gone, damaged, or different. I am going to have to rebuild myself and my life one brick at a time."

❧

These are some tips for the immediate aftermath of treatment:

- Remember that physical recovery is a process that will take approximately as long as the total duration of your treatment. Emotional recovery takes even longer. You cannot rush it.

- Be gentle on yourself. Ease your standards and lower your expectations.

- Anticipate that your friends and family will expect you to be right back to normal.

- Consider taking a few days or even weeks off from work. Use this break as a marker: the end of treatment and the beginning of the rest of your recovery.

- If feasible, plan a special vacation.

- Try to avoid stressful events or situations. Pay attention to your instincts and excuse yourself from such responsibilities.

- Do something indulgent: Have a facial, fill your house with flowers, spend the day with an old friend.

- Train yourself to never use the expression "my cancer." The cancer never was and certainly is not now part of you. Your blue eyes or your smile or your professional expertise are yours; your cancer is not. Instead, say "*the* cancer"—and note the difference.

- Make no important decisions. A life-threatening illness is a genuine opportunity to evaluate your life and your perspectives. This, however, is *not* the time to act on any of the ideas this evaluation may generate.

- Consider keeping a journal of your thoughts and feelings.

- Identify a few people you can really talk to about how you are feeling. Talk, talk more, and talk even more about it. Bottling up these feelings will not serve you well in the long run.

- If you have been thinking about doing so anyway, this is a wonderful time to bring home a pet. No one who believes she is about to die adopts a kitten or a puppy. By doing so, you are voting for life and bringing love into your days.
- If you cannot bring home a pet, plant a tree!

4

Physical Recovery

No one can tell you exactly how long it will take before this happens. I can promise you that it will happen but that it will take longer than you expect and much longer than you wish. Each week will be slightly easier than the one before, but you will continue to experience days of exhaustion, impatience, and depression.

Like emotional recovery, physical recovery occurs gradually over time. Obviously the specifics of your treatment and the overall quality of your health prior to diagnosis have much to do with how long this will take. Women who have undergone a bone-marrow or stem-cell transplant will certainly require much more time than women who have had "only" surgery and radiation therapy. Younger women are likely to feel better faster than older women, but there are certainly exceptions to all this. Susan, a social worker in her late thirties, participated in a biathlon ("It was a small biathlon," she insisted) while she was still on chemotherapy. I have also known women who biked the length of Cape Cod or ran a 10K road race during their treatment, but these are definitely the exceptions. Most women come to the end of their treatment feeling depleted.

When you look in the mirror, the woman looking back won't be the "you" you know and love. She looks different, and everything about her body feels different. Chances are you have either gained or lost weight, have lost some muscle tone and stamina, and have a much lower than normal energy level. And, if you had chemotherapy, these changes usually seem minor compared to the baldness and loss of other body hair! The loss of the hair on your head is the most obvious and public, but many women feel even worse about the absence of pubic hair and eyebrows and eyelashes.

Post-Surgery Changes

The biggest change from breast surgery, of course, is the change in your breast. Even if you were treated by a wide excision (also called a lumpectomy or partial mastectomy) rather than by a mastectomy, it is likely that your breast looks and feels different. Learning to live with your new body means, most of all, learning to live with your changed breast or reconstructed breast or absence of a breast. It is impossible to make sweeping statements about the reactions of women to these changes or about the importance of breasts to each of us. There is a very wide range in the value women ascribe to their breasts. Some have taken special pride in the beauty or size of their breasts, while others have treasured their natural function in nursing babies. Some women have never much liked their breasts, and I have actually known a few who felt more comfortable in their bodies after having bilateral mastectomies. Others have opted for immediate reconstruction following mastectomy and have totally new breasts. The point is that we are all different, and your own feelings, whatever they are, are important and must be understood and respected. Sometimes there are surprises, as women who felt that they could never live without a breast find that it doesn't matter so much after all, while others who did not expect to care find that they are miserable until they have reconstruction. By this time, you have had some months to begin to adjust to whatever your breast now looks like.

If you had a mastectomy without immediate reconstruction, you may gradually become comfortable living without a breast. You may adapt to wearing a prosthesis or you may decide to meet the world on your own new terms. It is possible to dress in ways that camouflage the fact that half of your chest is flat. Jackets and loose cardigans, long draped scarves, and vests may be successful. Without a prosthesis, it is harder to hide the fact during warmer weather or if you prefer close-fitting sweaters or shirts.

If you decide that you are unhappy living without a breast, you can consult a plastic surgeon about reconstruction at any time. Reconstructive surgery can be done years after a mastectomy. It is also sometimes possible to have partial reconstruction to improve the cosmetic result of a lumpectomy. The cosmetic result of reconstructive surgery is highly variable and depends upon numerous factors: the size and location of the tumor, the type of reconstruction, the way in which your body heals, the skill of the surgeon, the size of your breast.

If you consider breast reconstruction, it is important to talk with women who have had this surgery. As is true with any medical or surgical procedure, you will hear different reports from patients than from doctors. Ask them about their overall satisfaction with the result, about the recovery period, about any problems they have had, and whether they would make the same choice again. Specifically ask if they would work again with the same plastic surgeon. It is likely that some of these women will offer to show you their reconstructed breast. Say yes. Looking at the real thing is different than looking at pictures.

Be aware that there are widely diverse outcomes from breast reconstruction. Some women are very satisfied with their new breasts; some are even pleased by them. Some women have commented on having a "perky sixteen-year-old breast" while the other breast is sagging in an age-appropriate way. Others are disappointed in the appearance or experience chronic discomfort or pain from the surgery. The pain, in these cases, is generally not in the breast but in the part of the body (either the back or the abdomen) where muscle and tissue were moved. Sometimes women describe a permanent sensation of constriction, like a too-tight bra, around their upper body. I have also known a few women who bitterly regretted having had reconstruction either because of a bad cosmetic outcome or, worse, because of chronic physical problems resulting from the procedure. Ask the plastic surgeon to show you pictures of his less-than-perfect outcomes. Talk with women who are satisfied as well as some who are not.

Anticipate that a reconstructed breast will function very well as a "fashion accessory," enabling you to worry less about what you wear and to be more comfortable with your appearance. However, a reconstructed breast will never look exactly like a natural breast and it will always lack sensation. To a partner's hand, it may seem the same. While you will feel nothing physically, you may feel quite a lot emotionally about this fact.

If you are considering reconstruction because you think that your husband or partner will be happier with your body or because you are single and think it will make meeting someone easier, think carefully and think long before proceeding. The only good reason for breast reconstruction is because *you* want the surgery and *you* believe you will feel more whole. Any kind of breast reconstruction means serious surgery with no guaranteed result. Most women who have reconstruction are glad they did, but some do find that they manage perfectly well without it.

There are other minor post-breast-surgery changes that affect most women. Many of these aftereffects are the result of the axillary surgery that removes some lymph nodes in the armpit. If you had the more recently used sentinel-node biopsy procedure (a less invasive surgery), you will probably have fewer of these reactions. But whichever nodal procedure you had, you may have an area of numbness on the back of your arm or your armpit. You may feel some tightness or discomfort when you raise your arm over your head. Some women have more significant difficulty with range of motion or, in extreme cases, have a frozen shoulder. If you feel that you are limited in the movement of your arm on the surgery side, it is a good idea to consult with a physical therapist who is experienced in working with women who have had breast surgery. See her sooner rather than later, because earlier intervention makes a big difference in outcome.

Post-Radiation Changes

If you have had radiation therapy, it is important that you speak with your radiation oncologist or nurse about what physical changes to anticipate in the following weeks and months. Radiation continues to actively work in the area of your body that was treated for a while after the treatment itself ends, so your skin may continue to become redder and more blistered. If this happens, you can safely use the creams and soap you were directed to use during the weeks of radiation therapy. You might also try goat's milk soap if your skin feels tender. Jessica, a large-breasted woman who suffered quite serious and painful burns from her radiation treatment, found that she was most comfortable in a warm bath. She laughed that the rest of her skin turned prunelike in the water while her sore breasts floated comfortably.

If you had a "boost"—extra radiation targeted to only the tumor bed, the immediate area where the tumor was located—that part of your breast is likely to become redder and more burned after the treatment has been completed. Since a boost is given at the end of a course of radiation, the consolation is that the rest of your breast and the entire radiated area will be healing and improving even if the boost area itself is worse. In general, it is reassuring how quickly your breast will heal. Most women, of course, finish radiation with some degree of redness and tenderness on their treated breast. It is often described as being similar to a sunburn. A few, however, do end up with more-serious burns that take longer to heal.

Your treated breast may always be slightly darker in color than it was prior to the radiation. The texture of the skin might also be slightly different. The normal swelling that accompanies radiation therapy can take up to a year to disappear, so you may not really know how large or small your breast will be for many months. Women who were radiated in the 1970s and early 1980s were sometimes left with very hard breast tissue. Fortunately, the technology has greatly improved, so this is no longer a problem. Radiation does leave the scar tissue from the surgery more firm, and it may take a while for you to become familiar with the changed feel of that part of your breast. Over time, sometimes years, the scar tissue is likely to soften.

You may also experience shooting nervelike pains in your breast and down your arm. These are due to the gradual healing of nerves that were severed during your surgery, and radiation can make them worse. After treatment, some women also report that an ache in their treated breast, armpit, and arm is worse during damp weather. This is normal.

Sometimes, approximately six months after finishing radiation, women find that their breast suddenly becomes quite red again. This is called "radiation recall" and is almost always no more than an alarming nuisance. If this happens, you probably will want to call your radiation oncologist to sort out what is happening and to rule out the possibility of an infection. Do not be overly alarmed; it is not unusual and will quickly improve.

Weight Gain

The fact that many women gain weight on chemotherapy comes as a shock to most of us! Having cancer is usually associated with weight loss, and it seems a bitter and ironic twist that undergoing chemotherapy may result in a gain of ten to twenty pounds. While there is some controversy about the reasons for the weight gain, there appear to be two primary causes. The first is that the chronic low-level nausea is often somewhat controlled by frequent snacks and nibbling. If you munched on crackers or popcorn or even fruit pretty continuously for six months, it is likely that you took in more calories than your body burned. A more frequent cause is the change in metabolism brought about by the combination of chemotherapy and, often, a chemically induced menopause. While postmenopausal women generally weigh more than younger women, most of them gain those pounds slowly over the course of several years.

Chemotherapy-induced menopause occurs abruptly, which means that the additional pounds are also gained more quickly. In addition, most women in chemotherapy are less physically active than normal, so it is likely that they burn fewer calories in exercise or even in the course of normal daily activities. Weight gain, usually in the five-to-fifteen-pound range, is also a known side effect of tamoxifen and other hormonal therapies.

As we all know, excess weight increases the risk of

other health problems: diabetes, hypertension, heart disease, and strokes. In addition, extra weight may mean more estrogen in your body, while reduced estrogen levels are preferable for women who have had breast cancer. In postmenopausal women, estrogen can be produced by fat cells. (In premenopausal women, this is also true, although the dominant producer of estrogen is obviously the ovaries.) In theory, therefore, those of us who are hoping to minimize the estrogen in our bodies may be concerned about extra pounds. This is the reason that you may sometimes read that being overweight—that is, having lots of fat cells—is a risk factor for breast cancer.

Every woman knows the pressures in our society to be thin; many of us spent years struggling with diets long before we had breast cancer. Unfortunately, it seems to be true that it is even harder to lose weight after breast cancer treatment than it was before. Whether this is due to the normal metabolic changes brought about by menopause or by the chemotherapy itself is unknown, but it hardly matters why. What does matter is that you are probably going to have to work even harder to lose weight.

Weight loss is one of the most common concerns in my post-treatment support groups. Whenever it comes up, there is much animated discussion and much laughter. The group consensus is that feeling fat seems even worse after breast cancer because you are also likely to be feeling less attractive, desirable, and womanly than usual. When coupled with the growing-in hair and the lackluster self-image of most women freshly out of treatment, the excess pounds feel terrible. The women I know have tried all kinds of diets in an attempt to lose this unwelcome weight. Sometimes some variant of the high-protein low-carbohydrate plan works fairly well. Other women have successful experiences at Weight Watchers and similar group programs. Exercise always makes a difference. Most of us gradually manage to lose much, but not all, of the added weight. It seems to be a fact of life after breast cancer that you will probably weigh five to ten pounds more than you did before you were diagnosed.

As Libby said, "Would you rather be thin and dead or fatter and alive?" Put in that context, there is no question that additional weight is a very small price to pay for good health. Learning to feel comfortable in your skin and attractive in your body takes time. Try hard not to be self-critical about how different you think you look than you did two years ago. Believe the people around you who say that you look great. Tell yourself over and over that you are healthy and strong and will soon look better than ever.

One unexpected benefit is that most women who have had cancer rapidly get over their issues about aging. When you are most worried about living, it is not so hard to be thankful to be fifty or sixty or older. The extra pounds or wrinkles or sags seem relatively unimportant when you are grateful to be alive to have them.

The secret is coming to terms with your new body and learning to be at home in it (and this is true whether you are thinking about added weight or different hair or the loss or change of a breast). Life is too short to subsist solely on carrot sticks, and most of us decide that our enjoyment of food is part of our new appreciation and zest for life.

Tips for Weight Loss:

- Avoid crash diets. The weight may come off, but it will almost certainly come back on.
- The basic plan is "Eat less and exercise more."
- Exercise does not have to mean time at the gym or out jogging. Explore ways to burn some calories that can be easily incorporated into your day. For example, park a little farther from the store or take the stairs rather than the elevator; instead of driving, walk on short errands.
- Think in terms of weekly intake rather than what you eat during a single day. This makes it less guilt-inducing if you splurge and more likely that you will cut back the following day to balance your intake.
- Allow yourself treats. Just remember that they are "treats" and not the daily norm.
- Move clothes that are too small to the back of your closet or even into another room. It is too depressing every morning to look at the waistline you cannot zip or the blouse you cannot button.
- Work on moderation and balance. You have come through a major life crisis and are committed now to fully appreciating and enjoying your life. You will not be happy if you think you are fat, but neither will you be happy if you never eat the foods you love.

Hair

As hard as it is to be bald during chemotherapy, it is harder still to be bald when you are finished. Hair loss is so publicly associated with the role of the cancer patient that we are all frantically eager to have our hair back the minute the treatment is over. The unfortunate fact is that hair grows an average of half an inch per month. Remember that your body won't even realize that you are done with treatment until the day comes and goes when, if you were still receiving chemotherapy, it would have been time to go in for your next treatment. Remember, too, that your hair begins its growth inside your scalp and must grow for some time before you can even discern stubble. Most women see fuzz on their heads six to eight weeks after their final chemotherapy. In general, most women are not comfortable going without a wig or hat or scarf until three or four months have elapsed since their final chemotherapy. Unless you kept your hair very short, it is likely to take an additional three or four months to gain enough length to have the style you had before cancer.

You have probably heard and seen that the hair usually tends to come in curly. Even if your hair was always stick-straight, you may have little ringlets for several months. Some women describe their hair as looking like a lamb's or a poodle's. As the hair grows, its increasing length and weight often pull out the curls so they gradually become waves. However, some women's hair stays curly forever. Conversely, others end up with hair that is straighter than their precancer hair. The early hair growth is likely to feel baby-fine, but the texture will become more adultlike before long. Finally, the color may be different. No one really knows why these changes occur. Many women say, laughing, that they have colored their hair for so long that they really don't know what its natural color would be. Growing-in hair may be more or less gray than you remember. I have known a few women whose new hair completely changed— red and curly instead of light brown and straight, or dark brown and straight instead of dark blond and wavy. Caroline liked her red wig so much that she ended up coloring her regrown hair red rather than the blond she was accustomed to. Meredith decided to stop coloring her hair altogether and to enjoy the freedom of her gray curls. Elaine could not wait to be blond again and had her inch-long new gray hair dyed as soon as her hairdresser said there was enough to manage the job. Whatever your new hair looks like, you will be delighted to have it. As Judith said, "There is no such thing as a bad hair day when you have hair!"

Eyebrows and eyelashes grow back quickly. You will probably want to begin shaving your legs and armpits in a month or six weeks. Remember that the armpit of your treated side may stay numb. In that case, take extra care as you shave, because you will not feel a nick. Your pubic hair will also come back quickly and may be either sparser or much more luxuriant than it was before.

Tips for the Growing-In Period

- Plan on it taking three to four months before you are comfortable being out without something covering your head. Don't frustrate yourself by hoping for an impossible schedule.
- Consider the possibility of being comfortable with a far shorter haircut than you might ever have chosen. Some people even consider it chic!

- Daily intake of brewer's yeast (a vitamin B complex) may hasten hair growth. Make sure that you buy tablets, not powder, which has a strong and unpleasant taste.
- Massaging your scalp in the shower every day, with or without lotion or conditioner, may encourage hair growth.
- Buy a few new hats and scarves to wear during this period. You will tire very quickly of the ones you wore during chemotherapy.
- When you think your hair is still too short to be seen in public, try going somewhere where you are a stranger. You may well find that no one notices your short hair or that you are even complimented on its style.
- It is medically safe to color your hair, if you wish, as soon as it is long enough for this to be feasible. There is no truth to the rumors that hair dye causes cancer.
- Remember your sense of humor! When asked where she had gotten her very short and chic haircut, Wendy answered, "At the Beth Israel Deaconess Medical Center."

Lymphedema

Lymphedema, or swelling of the arm or hand, can happen after the removal of underarm lymph nodes during breast cancer surgery. Anyone who has had a mastectomy or a lumpectomy as well as axillary dissection is at risk. If you have also had radiation therapy that included the underarm area, the risk is slightly greater. When lymph nodes have been removed during surgery (and even if ten or fifteen or more were removed, plenty are left behind), drainage from some of the lymphatics—the fine channels that drain lymph into the bloodstream——may be impaired by scarring, causing the arm and possibly the hand to swell. Lymphedema was more common in the past, when more-radical surgeries removed more of the underarm lymph nodes. There are widely varying estimates, ranging from 5 percent to 33 percent, of the number of women who eventually develop lymphedema after breast surgery. It can happen from days to even years after surgery and can be caused by infection, trauma (injury), strenuous exercise, heavy weight bearing, or by the air pressure changes during a long airplane trip, as well as by unknown factors.

Several women I know who are living with lymphedema have decided that, even though it cannot be cured, it can be managed and incorporated into their lives. There may even be balances and trade-offs you can make. Sandy's identity as an athlete is very important to her. Even when she suddenly developed lymphedema, she decided that playing golf and riding her bicycle for long distances were more vital to her sense of well-being than a completely normal and slender arm. She therefore has chosen to live with wearing a pressure sleeve, nightly massage, and periodic swelling and discomfort. Someone else might make a different decision and change certain habits or activities. Once again, it is important to remember that you do have some choices and some control over your decisions.

You may hear that lymphedema is a high-protein edema, meaning that there is protein in the lymph fluid, but decreasing your protein intake will not affect this. In fact, a diet too low in protein may weaken the connective tissue and make any lymphedema worse. For this and other health reasons, it is important to eat a balanced diet with low sodium, plenty of fiber, and adequate protein.

Lymphedema is uncomfortable and, depending on its degree, can be quite unsightly. It can come and go but, once you have experienced it, it is likely to recur. It can be treated by wearing pressure sleeves or gloves, by massage or physical therapy, or by using special pumps that drain the fluid. If you experience even minimal lymphedema, it is wise to consult with a physical therapist who is experienced in working with women who have had breast surgery. Earlier treatment will maximize the odds of successful intervention. Since there is no real cure for lymphedema, it makes sense to follow some precautions to try to prevent it. It also makes sense to not obsess about the possibility. Lymphedema can happen, but it usually doesn't, and it would be a mistake to let your concerns become a major worry in your life.

Lymphedema Precautions:

- Wear gloves when you garden or work outdoors.
- Wear gloves if you are working with strong detergents or other chemicals.
- Avoid cutting cuticles on your affected side. In general, it is fine to have manicures, but ask the manicurist to gently push back, not cut, your cuticles. The reason for not cutting the cuticles on the affected side is to avoid the risk of an infection. Infection is a possibility if manicurists do not adequately sterilize their scissors and nippers between clients. In less careful, high-volume operations, even pushing back the cuticles may be risky—if done a

bit roughly, it can break the skin. If you do have professional manicures, choose your manicure salon and your
manicurist carefully and express your concerns to her.

- If you have a cut, scrape, burn, or bite on your affected
  hand or arm, wash it, apply antibiotic ointment, and cover
  it with a Band-Aid. It is wise to carry antibiotic ointment
  with you when you travel.

- Avoid tight sleeves, cuffs, or jewelry on that arm and
  hand.

- Be sensible about your exercise routine. If you have any
  doubts, consult with your surgeon or a physical therapist. Do not overtire your affected arm. If it starts to
  ache, stop whatever you are doing and elevate it.

- Do not carry heavy bags or suitcases with that arm. The
  motion to be avoided is the straight-arm position, with
  the weight hanging from your hand (i.e., the way you
  normally carry a suitcase). Do not lift more than fifteen
  pounds with that arm. Try to get into the habit of carrying things with your other arm.

- Use an electric razor, or at the very least shave very carefully under that arm.

- If you already have swelling, wear a pressure bandage or
  sleeve when you fly. Drink extra fluids on the plane.
  Some lymphedema experts suggest that *all* women who
  have had breast surgery that included the removal of axillary nodes wear a pressure sleeve when they fly. This
  becomes a personal decision, since you must balance the
  inconvenience and mild discomfort of wearing such a
  sleeve against its possible preventive value. A more comfortable compromise position might be to wrap your arm
  with an Ace bandage; this will provide some protection

during long flights. You can also try to keep it somewhat elevated.

- Do not allow an injection, an IV, or blood to be drawn from the affected arm unless there is no alternative. If you have had bilateral surgeries this cannot be avoided, but in that case make sure that your health-care provider is aware of your cancer-surgery history.

- Whether or not you have lymphedema, you will need to be extra alert for the following signs of infection: redness, tenderness, swelling, warmth, or fever. *If you experience any of these symptoms, call your doctor right away.* You may need to start taking antibiotics immediately to prevent a serious infection. Do not minimize or underreact to any of these symptoms. The situation can change and worsen very quickly.

- These lymphedema precautions must be followed for the rest of your life.

Cardiac Complications

If you received Adriamycin as part of your chemotherapy, you will have been told that cardiac toxicity, causing heart-muscle damage, can be one of the long-term side effects. The doses of Adriamycin used for adjuvant breast cancer chemotherapy are well below the doses that cause cardiac damage. As an additional precaution, you probably had tests before beginning chemotherapy to be sure that you had no heart problems. Very few women who receive this chemotherapy drug experience any kind of treatment-related heart trouble in the future.

However, I have known two women who developed

cardiac difficulties within two years of their chemotherapy. In both cases, they had a preexisting cardiac condition and, in retrospect, might have been better served with a different drug regimen. Cancer is frightening, and heart disease is also frightening. The combination can be overwhelming. If you experience any kind of chest pain or shortness of breath or dizziness, call your doctor. If you ever find yourself in a doctor's office or an emergency room where you are not known, make sure that you mention you have received Adriamycin in the past.

Fatigue and Low Energy

You are impatient to return to your old life, and to do this requires that you feel well and strong. To repeat yet again, it will take as long as the total duration of your treatment to feel really well, although you will feel better with each passing week. Your body has been through a great deal and it needs time and rest to recover. As you know, chemotherapy and radiation kill many healthy cells along with the cancerous ones, so your body will be expending energy toward healing itself.

As has been true every step along the way, each woman is different and will regain her energy level at her own pace. It does not help to push it. Your pretreatment physical condition, your age, and your treatments all affect how quickly you recover. You are likely to require more sleep and more unstructured time than usual for quite a while. You may experience multiple hot flashes during the night that awaken you and may even require a change of nightgowns. If you stay out late a couple of nights in a row, you will feel it. If you need to put in several consecutive long workdays, you will notice it. You may decide that certain events or obligations are worth the fatigue afterward, but be prepared for it.

Long-term fatigue following treatment can be debilitating and frightening. It is all too easy to interpret your lack of energy as a sign that the cancer is back or that you are not well. If you find that your fatigue persists beyond the "as long as your treatment" rule, it can be helpful to consider your total lifestyle. Perhaps you are not sleeping well, not eating in a healthy fashion, trying to cram too much into every twenty-four hours, or struggling with many unresolved feelings. I would suggest that your first step be to think about those feelings. Many women who have carried on normally and sturdily through the months of treatment have not allowed themselves to acknowledge them. Although this may have been a useful defense mechanism or coping tool during treatment, it may be tripping you up now. Anxiety and sadness can be interfering with sleep, whether by keeping you awake or by giving you nightmares. Psychological struggle definitely saps your energy. It is of paramount importance that you now find a place and a way to process the intense emotions that are associated with the diagnosis and treatment of breast cancer.

Many women plan a vacation to mark the end of their breast cancer treatment. It can be wonderful during the months of treatment to read travel guides and consider the possibilities. It helps to look forward, to remember that the treatments will end and life will continue. A vacation, even a few days away, can serve as an important marker. The cancer and all that came with it stand "before"; the rest of your life is "after."

If you are considering such a trip, remember that you do not yet have your normal stamina and physical strength. Even if you are accustomed to very active vacations, this may or may not be what you need now. Linda, a fund-raiser for a major charitable organization, always liked adventure travel. She could not imagine a vacation that did not include lots of physical activity and even physical challenges. A month after completing her radiation therapy, still bald from her chemotherapy, she took a rafting and camping trip through the Grand Canyon. This seemed relatively tame to her, although most of the women in her group were astounded by her choice of so active a trip. I, on the other hand, wanted nothing more than to lie on a beach and read after my own treatment ended, and that is exactly what I did.

Tips for Managing Fatigue

- Lower your expectations and remember that this, too, will pass.
- Continue some of the energy-saving tricks you learned during your treatments. It is still fine to bring in take-out food, ask your friends to sometimes take your day of carpool driving, or hire someone to clean your house.
- Think of your energy in terms of a savings account. You have a set amount, although with time it is appreciating. Spend it wisely.
- Pay attention to your energy swings during the day. If you are more energetic in the morning, for example, try to schedule your tasks then.
- Lie down during the afternoon. Even if you don't sleep, your body will rest.

- Get into bed half an hour earlier than you think you are ready to sleep. You may find that you are nodding off only a few pages into your book. If not, you will be relaxed—and have more time to read than usual.
- Resume an exercise program when you can. Moderate exercise will help you feel more energetic. Walking can be particularly helpful and is relatively easy to incorporate into your day.

Hot Flashes

Although we all understand that hot flashes are not a medical problem, they can be an enormous personal problem. Women who have been treated for breast cancer may experience particularly intense hot flashes because of the abrupt transition to menopause. Instead of a gradual perimenopause, their periods can stop after a single chemotherapy treatment. Women who had been taking hormone-replacement therapy (HRT) must stop at once, so they, too, may experience intense menopausal symptoms. Younger women who maintain their periods through their treatments may later opt for oophorectomy (surgical removal of their ovaries) or be given hormonal treatment to suppress ovulation and estrogen. In any of these instances, hot flashes may become a major problem.

Be reassured that they will eventually diminish in both frequency and intensity and will later stop. There is enormous variability in that intensity. You may find, as I did, that they are most often "warm" rather than "hot" flashes and easily managed. However, you may find that your sleep is interrupted many times each night, that you are suddenly beet red and glistening with sweat during the day, and that your quality of life is truly compromised. The management of hot flashes is discussed more fully in the chapters on complementary therapies, sexuality, and hormonal therapies. The bottom line is that there is no one strategy that will help every woman all of the time. Your best bet is to experiment and to talk with other women about what may have helped them.

The two basic approaches to managing hot flashes are medicinal and behavioral. Since you have had breast cancer, you cannot take HRT. Charles Loprinzi, M.D., of the Division of Medical Oncology at the Mayo Clinic, has devoted extensive research to the treatment of hot flashes with a variety of medications, both prescription and herbal or complementary. Dr. Loprinzi has found that most of the alternatives help some women for a while, but none helps everyone, and all lose most of their effectiveness over time. Ask your doctor whether he thinks medication is advisable; he will know which drug may be appropriate for you.

There are also nonprescription and herbal remedies that are often suggested for the treatment of hot flashes. Again, this is discussed more fully in Chapter 7. Remember that over-the-counter drugs are still drugs, even though they do not require a prescription to purchase. Err on the side of caution and talk first with your doctor before trying them. Many herbal treatments are helpful for hot flashes because they contain plant estrogens (isoflavones or phytoestrogens), so they may be dangerous for women who have had breast cancer. Any of these herbal remedies should be used with caution and care and *only after* a prior discussion with your doctor.

Soy is frequently mentioned as a possible treatment for hot flashes and other menopausal symptoms. Again, this is a subject of much controversy and must be discussed with your doctor. Some physicians are concerned about soy consumption because soy is rich in plant estrogens. Therefore it seems prudent to never take soy capsules or powder or to drink soy milk in large quantities without talking first with your doctor.

Behavioral and lifestyle interventions begin with careful attention to your own life and hot-flash patterns. Are there particular situations or times of day when you know that you are apt to have more or more-intense hot flashes? Stress is a known trigger, and some women find that spicy foods, caffeine, or alcohol also brings them on. Other candidates are any situation that raises your body temperature: hot baths or showers, hot tubs, hot rooms, hot weather.

So what might help? Exercise tops the list of positive behaviors. Not only is regular exercise likely to reduce your hot flashes, it will also help with many other issues, including weight, mood swings, and bone density. Since stress always makes flashes worse, you now have an additional incentive to try to reduce the stress in your life. In addition to avoiding stressful situations as much as you can, learn some relaxation techniques or deep breathing.

Practical tips for hot flashes abound among women who are living with breast cancer. Suggestions include:

- Keep ice water with you during the day and in a carafe by your bed at night.

- Keep a previously frozen wet washcloth in a small cooler by your bed. If you awaken drenched and hot in the middle of the night, it will be soothing.
- Keep a few extra pillows near your bed. Changing to a fresh and cool one will help.
- Avoid synthetic sheets. Use only cotton and cotton flannel.
- If you share your bed, consider not sharing all of your covers. Either use two sets of blankets or look for an electric blanket that has two settings, one for each side.
- If you don't already have one, put an air conditioner in your bedroom. You may find you want to use it all year.
- Dress in layers. This is probably the single most important tip. Dressing in natural fibers will also help. Avoid turtlenecks.
- Buy a few paper fans and keep them in your office and at home. Look for them in Asian stores.
- Consider a small handheld battery fan. You may feel ridiculous holding it near your face, but it will feel wonderful!

Muscle Stiffness and Joint Pain

Many women report some degree of muscle stiffness and joint pain following treatment for breast cancer, especially after chemotherapy. Arthritis is not uncommon among women who have had chemotherapy for breast cancer. It is never possible to know whether arthritis would have happened anyway, but, like so many things, it often seems to develop suddenly. This can be especially bad upon awakening in the morning, and you may feel one hundred years old as you first get out of bed. Other times when the stiffness is likely to be worse are after a long car or plane trip or even after sitting in one position at work.

Some women report that swimming, yoga, and gentle stretches help. An over-the-counter dietary supplement containing glucosamine and chondroitin helps many women with stiffness and aches. It certainly won't hurt you, so it is probably worth a try. If you are feeling especially uncomfortable, a warm bath can be soothing. Make sure that you have a firm and comfortable mattress. And as in so many other matters, your best coping strategy may involve your sense of humor. If you can find a way to laugh or at least smile at your awkwardness, it is likely to pass before you stop grinning.

Patricia Ganz, M.D., and her colleagues at UCLA studied more than eight hundred breast cancer survivors and asked about their symptoms between one and five years after the completion of their treatments. The top ten reported symptoms were:

1. general aches and pains: 70 percent
2. unhappiness with appearance of body: 69 percent
3. muscle stiffness: 64 percent
4. forgetfulness: 64 percent
5. joint pains: 62 percent
6. headaches: 59 percent
7. hot flashes: 55 percent
8. short temper: 53 percent
9. early awakening: 52 percent
10. breast sensitivity: 51 percent*

*Ganz et al., 1998, *Journal of Clinical Oncology*, 16, 501–514.

Obviously, several of these symptoms are likely to be frightening. It is difficult, especially in the early months, to experience any physical ache or pain, even a twinge, with any objectivity; they seem to be announcing the spread of your cancer.

Many oncologists operate by the "two-week rule." This means that any pain that disappears in two weeks or less is so minor that you do not even need to mention it at your next visit, much less call in a panic. If a pain persists for longer than two weeks, however, you should call your doctor, even though the overwhelming majority of such worries turn out to be unfounded. If, of course, you are so frightened by a pain that you are unable to sleep or to concentrate on your daily responsibilities, go ahead and call your doctor. It is always better to be reassured than to suffer. Once again, time helps, and you will gradually become more comfortable with your body.

Memory Problems

The expression *chemobrain* is used over and over to describe intellectual and memory problems following chemotherapy: the general blunting of mental sharpness, fuzziness with quantitative thinking, and common difficulties with short-term memory, especially with finding words. I have even known two accountants who were forced to make professional changes when they found they could not perform as well as they had previously.

It was, therefore, both reassuring and disheartening when Tim A. Ahles, Ph.D., a psychologist, presented a study at an American Cancer Society meeting in March of

2000. Conducted at the Dartmouth Medical School, the study followed seventy-one patients who were cancer-free, following chemotherapy for breast cancer or lymphoma, for an average of ten years, as compared with fifty-eight patients, also cancer-free, who had been treated with radiation and/or surgery. Overall, in the nine areas of cognitive functioning that were measured, those who had chemotherapy scored significantly lower than those who did not. Although the majority were still thinking clearly, between one-quarter and one-third of those tested scored near the bottom in at least four of the categories. Only half as many of the radiation or surgery patients fared this poorly.*

Ahles's study does leave us with mixed feelings. It is helpful to learn that, yes, indeed, the intellectual changes you are experiencing are real and are related to the treatments, especially chemotherapy, that you have had. On the other hand, it is discouraging that the people whom he studied were still experiencing cognitive changes ten years after their treatment finished. It is also impossible to differentiate between such changes as a consequence of treatment and those that are normal changes due to aging. Still, on balance, it can be reassuring to know that any intellectual fuzziness that you are experiencing is a normal and expected consequence of what you have been through.

Since many of us are also concerned about Alzheimer's disease, problems with memory may make us worry about this even more. It is reassuring to differentiate between the

*These findings were published in the *Journal of Clinical Oncology* in January 2002 (Volume 20, 485–493).

cognitive troubles that are related to cancer treatment and normal aging vs. those that may be early signs of Alzheimer's. The primary symptom of very early Alzheimer's disease is difficulty remembering words or events from the immediate past. For example, someone with this problem might not recall a conversation she had ten minutes previously. This is very different from the memory and cognitive problems associated with chemobrain.

Most of us express frustration about these problems but find ways to adapt. The general sense is that while mental capacity does gradually improve with time, there is a real question as to whether it ever returns to pretreatment levels. In my groups, this is a common topic. We know that we are resilient and that brains can compensate and relearn. There is even new evidence that neural pathways can regenerate.

We may have to work a little harder to create new learning pathways in our brains. Here are tricks and strategies that may help.

- Read, read, read. Read anything and everything. You will find yourself widely and better informed; this is a huge confidence builder!
- Play games; ideally play games with nine- to thirteen-year-old children. Your experience and strategic skills will give you the edge over their sharp young memories.
- Find things to memorize. One woman joined a vocal group and had to memorize many songs for their performances; this was both fun and excellent mental exercise.

- Do crossword and other puzzles from the daily newspaper.
- Play bridge or chess.
- Keep a journal, and write short essays or even newsy letters or e-mails to your friends. Whatever the format, write.
- Look for new challenges at work or even consider a new career.
- Change your daily routines and find new ways of managing old responsibilities.
- Make sure that you get enough sleep.
- Consider purchasing a tiny tape recorder that you can carry in your purse or clip to the visor in your car. When you think of something you need to remember, tape it. This becomes the equivalent of making oral to-do lists.
- Finally, you can often fake it. If you can't remember a particular word, use another. If you can't remember someone's name, form your sentence a different way.

And take heart from Marilyn's comment: "I've noticed that in situations where I feel terribly embarrassed, those around me are just empathizing and feeling grateful it's not them! Once I realized that, I stopped fretting." And when you are worried about your brain being blasted out from chemotherapy, just ask yourself how comfortable were you ten years ago with the computer skills that you now take for granted. Recovery is possible.

Dental Problems

You may find that you are having more trouble with your

teeth than ever before. Women who have had chemotherapy may be at increased risk for decay and the resulting treatments of fillings, caps, crowns, and even root canals. There are two possible reasons for this. The first is that chemotherapy, especially in the large doses used in some high-risk breast cancer or other clinical trials, suppresses the output of the salivary glands. They may never return to normal function. Because there is less saliva circulating in the mouth, more tooth decay may be the result.

Michael J. Burnes, D.M.D., of Brookline, Massachusetts, also suggests another possible cause. When people are stressed, they sometimes grind their teeth at night. Tooth grinding may cause tooth cracks, fractures, or other problems.

It is therefore even more important that you now maintain a routine of twice-yearly cleanings and visits to your dentist. Few of us enjoy these visits, but all of us would prefer to have problems caught early.

Nails

If you had chemotherapy, you probably noticed that your nails became somewhat discolored, brittle, and perhaps sensitive. These unwelcome changes may not disappear when your treatment ends. If you can possibly afford to do so, have at least a couple of professional manicures. (Do remember to have your cuticles pushed, not clipped, as a way to avoid possible infection.) A licensed nail technician can suggest specific nail-care products that will help you. The regular use of hand creams, some kind of nail-strengthening polish, and attention to tears and snags will help. Nail polish covers up a multitude of sins and will probably improve the look of your hands.

All in all, it can seem discouraging and thoroughly unfair that treatment to save your life has left you with so many physical changes. Over time, many of these will diminish and you will adapt to those that do not. Breast cancer treatment is one thing—an important thing, to be sure, but just one thing—that has happened to your body. That body has mostly served you well, and it has gotten you through these past difficult months. The sense of being comfortable in your skin will grow as time passes and you have daily evidence of your return to robust good health.

5

Medical Follow-Up

Like it or not, you will be seeing all of your doctors—your surgeon, radiation oncologist, and medical oncologist—in follow-up for a very long time, if not for the rest of your life. In general, it makes sense to try to coordinate and spread your visits so that you are seeing one or another of them at different times. Different doctors have different follow-up schedules, but most will want to see you approximately a month after the conclusion of their part of your treatment and then every three or four months for several years. After approximately three years, most physical side effects of treatment are resolved and you will be feeling well. It is important to note that "well" will likely be a different level of wellness than you were accustomed to prior to your diagnosis. After three years, however, almost all women have adapted and adjusted to their new normal levels of energy, libido, physical strength, and general well-being.

Your doctors will want to see you both to assess your recovery and, even more importantly, to check on the cancer. The hope and intent, obviously, is that the cancer has been cured. The risk of recurrence decreases after three years, is lower still between five and ten years, and is still lower a decade beyond diagnosis. For this reason, many doctors will choose to meet with you less often after five years, and you may see any one doctor only every six months or even annually thereafter.

If for any reason you are not satisfied with the relationship and care you are receiving from one of your doctors, the time of transition to after-treatment care is a reasonable moment to consider making a change. Ideally you will find yourself able to discuss your discontent with the doctor; perhaps the issues can be resolved. It is obviously simpler to stick with the doctors who already know you and have been working with you through your treatment. However, it is essential to remember that these will be very long-term patient–doctor relationships and that the cancer is likely to remain your biggest health concern in the years ahead. It is vital that you feel comfortable and safe with your caregivers. If you do not feel that way, if one of your doctors does not answer your questions, respond empathetically to your concerns, or seem to consider your well-being paramount, it is time to consider a change.

If you decide that you need to make a change, you are in a better position to do so now than would have been the case immediately after diagnosis or during your treatment. At this point, your care can be transferred with no interruption in your treatment; equally important, you are feeling less anxious and better able to carefully consider your options. Talk to other women you know with breast cancer and ask about their doctors. Ask them if they feel completely comfortable and well cared for; ask them if they like the logistics of the practice and if they find that their needs are seen as important now that they have completed active treatment. It is perfectly acceptable to schedule an appointment to interview a surgeon or medical oncologist to determine if you like his or her style and manner.

It may also be that you have to make a change because of a change in your medical insurance or a move to another city. If you are moving, ask your doctor for a referral in your new home before you leave. Most oncologists have friends and colleagues across the country, and if you like your current doctor you are likely to feel comfortable with people she suggests. Be reassured that there are fine oncologists everywhere in the United States and that, over time, you will feel as safe with your new doctor(s) as you did with those who cared for you right after your diagnosis.

After working with several different specialists during your treatment, it can be hard to figure out who is now in charge of your health care. You will still need to see a gynecologist for annual examinations and Pap smears, as well as a primary-care physician, or PCP, for your normal health needs. You will find that now that there is cancer in your medical history, every complaint or symptom is taken more seriously. A recurrence of your cancer is often a part of the differential diagnosis—the possibilities that your doctor considers when a problem arises. It can be upsetting to learn that not only do you worry about every ache and pain, but your doctors do, too!

It would be a very good idea to have a conversation

with your PCP and with your medical oncologist about how to manage the concerns and questions that are certain to come up over the next months and years. Whom do you call if your back has been hurting? If you have a sore throat and a fever? They will help you think about which problems belong in which doctor's domain. Some women also have a personal preference about whom they call with a worry. It may feel less scary to call your PCP, because she is not the one always thinking about your cancer. Alternatively, it may seem more reassuring to call your oncologist and be told that your problem certainly has nothing to do with your breast cancer.

One of the true shocks of completing active treatment is the realization that there will never be an absolute way to be sure you are completely well and free of cancer. You have become accustomed to the care and the regular reassurances of your doctors and other caregivers. During treatment, you probably gave little thought to how they would continue to monitor your progress once that was over or how they could be confident that you were continuing to do well. Now you are face-to-face with the reality that there is no way to be certain you are fine.

There are two kinds of breast cancer recurrence: local (in the breast) or distant. As is discussed in Chapter 16, the greater worry is a distant recurrence. Breast cancer that comes back in the same breast where it started is treatable and potentially curable. Breast cancer that returns in another part of your body is treatable but not curable. The most common sites of breast cancer metastases are bone, lung, liver, lymph nodes (usually in the underarm or neck), or brain. A breast cancer recurrence in any of these places would still be breast cancer. That is, breast cancer that recurs in the lung is breast cancer in the lung, not lung cancer. Your doctor has probably advised you of symptoms to be aware of: bone pain, a cough that persists, shortness of breath, enlarged lymph nodes, pain in the right side of your abdomen (where your liver is), neurological symptoms, or a general sense of feeling unwell.

It is frightening to consider any of these possibilities and unsettling to recognize that many of them are also symptoms of garden-variety ailments. How do you know the difference? The reality is that you can't know at the beginning. Bone pain, for example, is hard to differentiate from muscle or tendon pain. Cancer bone pain, however, does not come and go, does not move around, and gradually gets worse. Pain that disturbs your sleep at night needs to be reported to your doctor.

What kind of follow-up can you expect, and what are your doctors looking for during their examinations? In 1997, the American Society of Clinical Oncology (ASCO) released guidelines, or standards of care, for breast cancer follow-up. Its objective was "to determine an effective, evidence-based post-treatment surveillance strategy for the detection and treatment of recurrent breast cancer. Tests are recommended only if they have an impact on the outcome (survival) specified by the American Society of Clinical Oncologists (ASCO) in their clinical practice guidelines." This means that their expert panel carefully examined and evaluated the findings of multiple well-designed studies in order to establish safe and reasonable standards of care.

Their summary recommendations include monthly breast self-examination, annual mammography of both the treated and the other breast, and a careful physical examination and oral medical history every three to six months for the first three years and then every six to twelve months. They specifically do not recommend the routine use of bone scans, chest X rays, liver ultrasounds, CAT scans, or even tumor markers (CEA and CA 27.29) as part of blood tests.

The bottom line is that less is as good as more in terms of testing and that, in almost all instances, finding a recurrent breast cancer or metastasis a little sooner because of a blood test or scan will not make a difference in the outcome. For example, if a blood test indicated a rising breast cancer marker in February and follow-up X rays and scans found a small bone metastasis, the treatment for this problem (radiation and/or chemotherapy) will likely be just as effective whether it was begun in February or several months later when bone pain brought the problem to light. In addition, a person's quality of life may be better if she does not know of a serious problem until it causes a symptom or a clinical concern.

This may seem counterintuitive, and it is important to understand the difference between the medical and the psychological realities and recommendations. As you know, breast cancer that has spread or metastasized outside of the breast (this does not include the axillary lymph nodes) is treatable but not curable. The horse is out of the barn. Any therapy that is recommended to treat metastatic breast cancer will be just as helpful if begun now or if begun a little later. The time that treatment for metastatic breast cancer is initiated does not affect overall survival. This explains why waiting to deal with a metastasis until it declares itself by causing a symptom does not compromise the long-term outcome. A number of well-done clinical trials reinforce this point.

There are exceptions to these recommendations, and some physicians do choose to follow their patients using more tests. There is further discussion about kinds of follow-up tests later in this chapter. During the first two or three years after the end of your treatment, when the risk of recurrence is highest, your doctor may opt for blood tests to check tumor markers or for other X rays or scans. Do talk with your doctor about common symptoms of recurrence and make sure you understand what you need to report.

If you were treated as part of a clinical trial, the study will have specific guidelines for your follow-up care that are likely to include blood tests and scans. If this is your situation, you will have already been informed about these tests and will be expecting them during the years ahead.

As has been said earlier, it is almost always equally safe and effective to wait to begin treatment for metastatic disease until a symptom has made the problem obvious. The only exceptions would be symptoms that are clearly very frightening or disruptive. If you suddenly see double, have other neurological symptoms, or develop severe, constant headaches, you would want to be in touch with your doctor. If you were so short of breath that you could not comfortably climb stairs or you noticed that your abdomen had expanded so that you looked six months pregnant, you would want to be in touch with your doctor. However, situations like these are very rare for women who have been well until the problem occurred. For most concerns, remember the two-week rule.

It is important to remember that follow-up appointments with your doctors and any tests that he or she recommends are likely to be stressful. No matter how well you are feeling and how much you have been able to push cancer worries away from the center of your mind, returning to the doctor or going for a mammogram will be anxiety-producing. Many women report how unhappily surprised they are to discover that simply walking into the doctor's waiting room makes them feel nauseated and anxious. As time passes, you will find these visits slightly easier, but even women who are eight or ten years past their breast cancer diagnosis tell me that they don't sleep well the night before their appointments and continue to worry that something will turn out to be wrong.

It may be helpful to reassure yourself that these worries are completely normal. Try to identify what you are most worried about. If you fear that your doctor will discover another lump in your breast or an enlarged lymph node, you can do a careful self-examination and be fairly certain there is nothing to be found. If you are most worried about blood tests, you might consider having your blood drawn a few days prior to your appointment so that the results will be ready when you meet with your doctor. It may also help to consider what will enable you to handle these difficult days. Is it better to stay scheduled and busy or to give yourself time to be alone and quiet? Does it help to take a friend with you to an appointment, or do you feel better going alone? Just as it was helpful to have someone with you during your treatments, it may be helpful now. A friend can help you remember the questions you have, recall what the doctor said, and in general be a comfort and companion if you are feeling upset.

While there is controversy about which tests, if any, should be part of regular breast cancer aftercare, the trend has been to do fewer, rather than more, routine scans or X rays, with the one major exception of annual mammograms.

There are a number of tests that are sometimes used. They include:

- Mammography: You are already familiar with this breast X ray and know that it often detects breast cancers long before they could be found by clinical exam or touch. You will still need mammograms every year. Some surgeons order mammograms of the treated breast every six months for the first two years. Otherwise, doctors do not suggest more-frequent mammograms for women who have had breast cancer; an annual one is adequate. If you have had a mastectomy and reconstruction, you will probably not have mammography on that breast, since there is little to no breast tissue left after this surgery, and most doctors feel that mammograms are not useful. However, you will need to continue with annual mammograms on your remaining breast.

- Breast Ultrasound: Again, you may be familiar with breast ultrasound from the time of your diagnosis. Ultrasound uses sound waves that become images of the part of your body being examined. Often used in parallel with mammography, an ultrasound can detect whether a lump is solid or fluid-filled. It cannot indicate with certainty whether a lump is cancerous.

- Breast MRI: Magnetic resonance imaging (MRI) uses magnetic fields, not the radiation used in X rays, to take pictures of the body. It is very useful for the close examination of many internal organs and is now being tested at some centers as a screening tool for breast cancer. But while MRI is very sensitive, it is not very specific, so there have been difficulties in interpreting the results of this breast imaging, and it is not yet known whether it will turn out to be a useful tool for routine and universal screening. It is being used more frequently in women who are at particularly high risk for developing breast cancer, but it is not proficient at picking up preinvasive cancers.

- PET Scan: PET (positron emission tomography) scan is another relatively recent diagnostic test that is sometimes used in cancer care. However, the radiological pictures produced by these scans are difficult to interpret, and abnormalities may be visualized that are impossible to identify. The resulting anxiety and possible need for biopsies are problematic. For these reasons, PET scans are not routinely advised by many doctors, although they may become more common in the future when there is more information and greater expertise regarding their interpretation.

- Chest X Rays: We are all familiar with chest X rays ordered for reasons that have nothing to do with breast cancer (e.g., checking for pneumonia or as a standard preoperative test). Since breast cancer can metastasize to the lung, these tests can be used to determine whether there is any sign of cancer in the lung. However, they are not recommended for routine screening and are ordered only when there is a symptom that causes concern.

- Bone Scans: You may have had a bone scan as part of your initial staging at the time of your diagnosis. After a radioactive isotope is injected into a vein, the body is scanned and areas of bone activity light up in the picture. There can be reasons other than cancer (such as arthritis or past injury) that result in suspicious bone scans, and in such cases the scan would be followed by an X ray of the area of concern. Bone scans are not recommended for routine follow-up. They are ordered if there is bone pain and concern about a possible bone metastasis.

- CAT Scans: Computerized axial tomography is a specialized X ray that provides a detailed layered view of a particular part of the body. CAT scans are used in breast cancer care to explore the possibility of a metastasis to a specific organ or region of the body. In the case of known metastatic disease, they are used to evaluate the cancer's shrinkage or growth in response to ongoing treatment.

- MRI: In addition to being tested as a screening tool, magnetic resonance imaging is more often used, like CAT scans, to determine whether breast cancer has spread or to assess the response to ongoing treatment in the case of known metastatic disease. Neither MRI nor CAT scans are part of routine follow-up care, with the exception of guidelines for follow-up in some clinical trials.

- Blood Tests: You will have had blood drawn as part of your routine physical care or for one or another reason all your life, and you had blood drawn frequently during your chemotherapy to check your blood counts. There are several blood tests that may be used in routine follow-up care:

1. CBC, or Complete Blood Count: This looks at the number of white cells, red cells, and platelets in your blood. Do not be alarmed if it takes many months after chemotherapy for your counts to return to normal levels. It is even possible that they may never regain their previous levels and may always be lower than average. You can be completely healthy and well with blood counts that are at the low end of the normal range.

2. Blood Chemistries: These may be ordered to measure the functioning of your kidneys and liver. You may hear the term *Liver Function Tests*, *Liver Panel*, or *Liver Screen* for tests that measure the levels of liver enzymes and bilirubin, which can indicate cancer or other problems in the liver. Other blood chemistries, not cancer-specific, study levels of chloride, electrolytes (sodium, potassium, bicarbonate), urea nitrogen, creatinine (kidney function), and calcium levels.

3. Cancer Markers: These are the blood tests that cause most of the anxiety associated with follow-up care. If there is active breast cancer somewhere in your body, the division and growth of those cells may throw off certain substances that can be measured in the blood. These markers include the CEA and the CA 15-3 (or CA 27.29). Unfortunately, these marker results are not always reliable. It is possible to have elevated markers that result from smoking or other benign conditions and no cancer, and to have normal markers in the pres-

ence of metastatic disease. I have known women who
were panicked by a finding of an elevated marker at a
routine appointment. When their blood was redrawn to
check the accuracy of the test, the results came back
normal. If this should happen to you, keep in mind the
real possibility that the first reading was a lab error, a
false positive, and that the second specimen will be
normal.

These markers are especially frightening because we
cannot see or know what is in our blood. Most of us obses-
sively examine our breasts and our bodies before our appointments. When we can't feel anything unusual, we can be
slightly more confident walking into the doctor's examination room. Martha, a fifty-year-old health-care consultant,
described her experience at her one-year checkup this way:
"My cancer measure is a blood test called a CEA, and when
I went to have my blood drawn, I cried. The phlebotomist
said, 'Why are you crying?' and I said, 'Because I am afraid
that my cancer has come back.' He said, in a strong French
Creole accent, 'We will overcome!' which I thought was a
wonderful thing to say.

"Then when I met with my oncologist, the *very first*
thing he had to say, even before 'Good morning, Martha,'
was my CEA number. Even though it was normal, I cried
again.

"I can say that now, three years after finishing my treatment, I have gotten much better. Now I only cry when I
see my oncologist and am a 'Very Brave Girl' when I am
with the phlebotomist. Especially since there are so many
folks getting their blood drawn at the same time who are

obviously in the midst of treatment, I feel especially strongly that I have to behave.

"Fear of return of cancer is primal. We don't even know it is lurking in our subconscious until something like a checkup brings it lunging to the surface like the Loch Ness monster. And most of the time, it is just about as real as the Loch Ness monster."

It is important for you to continue with monthly breast self-examinations. No one knows your body as well as you do, and you must become familiar with the way your breast(s) feel. It is my impression, based on many conversations with many women, that even women who were compulsive about self-examination before their cancer find it very hard to continue it now. This reluctance may be due to the intense fear of finding something amiss or to the fact that the affected breast feels quite different from the way it did before cancer. Scar tissue, especially after radiation, feels hard and bumpy and "weird." Nonetheless, you must find a way to examine yourself frequently enough to become accustomed to this new feel as normal, so you will know if something changes. You cannot count on your doctors, no matter how frequently you are being examined by one of them, to be wholly responsible for noticing any change.

Unfortunately, I have known women who found a second cancer in either the same or the other breast some years after treatment. In some of these cases, their doctors could not feel anything abnormal but wisely followed up on the woman's sense that something had changed. It was then that a mammogram or an ultrasound showed the cancer. Just as before, you will know your body and your breasts better than anyone else, and you are the one most responsible for yourself. Be your own best advocate. If your doctor is not listening to you, keep talking. Insist upon a biopsy if you are truly worried about a change in your breast.

Follow-up testing is a frequent topic of conversation in my support groups for women who have completed their active treatments. They usually break pretty evenly between those who ask for blood tests or doctor visits as often as possible and those who prefer to distance themselves as much as possible from their medical care. Some are reassured by the return of normal test results and word that "Everything seems fine." Others understand that even normal test results and a normal physical examination are not a guarantee that all is truly well and would prefer to "not know of trouble one day sooner than I have to."

You will gradually figure out what strategy is best for you. Remember that recurrent breast cancer will always declare itself and become impossible to ignore. You can choose to pursue less vigilant follow-up and be just as well as if you were opting for more-frequent visits and tests. Assuming that you are seeing your doctors every three to six months, doing breast self-examinations, paying attention to your body and how it feels, and having annual mammograms, what matters most is your psychological well-being. As time passes, you will discover what helps you to feel safer, and it is likely that your doctor will be glad to work with you in those ways that most enhance your sense of well-being.

If you ever have to cope with a recurrence of your breast cancer, it is probable that you will be the first to know. While doctors at follow-up visits do find some problems themselves, most symptoms are noticed by patients between visits. This is both the good news and the bad news. My husband, who is an experienced medical oncologist, tells his patients: "If you are feeling fine, all the odds are that you *are* fine." Be reassured by your own good health. But remain vigilant, even if this means that you, like most of us, become overaware of every ache and pain and must struggle to not become a hypochondriac in monitoring your body.

When I speak with women who have just completed treatment, I warn them that, especially in the first months or years, they will be convinced that every stiff neck or backache or headache is the cancer coming back. It is very likely that, over the course of the first post-treatment year, you will experience an ache or pain that frightens you enough to call your doctor. It can be even more frightening to discover that your call will be taken seriously and you will probably be seen quickly. Follow the two-week rule: For most concerns, if your pain or symptoms do not persist for two full weeks, you do not need to report them to your doctor. If it does last that long, you should call, but you should also keep it in mind that it is still likely to be of little consequence. As time passes and you live through several such incidents of fear and relief, you will be slightly less frightened when something feels wrong. It is easier to believe in a possible good outcome when you have been through that experience.

Approximately two years after my cancer diagnosis and a year and a half after completing treatment, my husband and I took a long-awaited and wonderful vacation in St. John. Basking in the sun and in the silken sea, I felt whole and well and completely healthy. But a few days after our return, while scratching my neck, I felt a hard lymph node. Instantly the clock stopped and rolled back. Once more it was a February morning, and once more, upon awakening, I felt a lump that terrified me. Once more I asked my husband to please feel this spot, and, just like the last time, his face turned ashen. Desperately reaching for any courage and wisdom I had found over the previous two years, I announced this was not going to spoil our Sunday morning and jumped out of bed to find my running clothes. Taking my lead and unsure how else to navigate the treacherous minutes, he followed suit.

There is a leash law in our community, and we tend to keep our own dog on a lead when we are running or walking on the streets. This morning, we encountered a woman running with her unleashed dog, who in a friendly fashion came to sniff and prance with our leashed Jasper and us. To my horror and astonishment, I found myself literally yelling at her: "Don't you know there is a leash law here? Put your dog on a leash right this minute!" I knew I was being ridiculous but I could not stop myself, and when my embarrassed husband tried to say something conciliatory, I, of course, snapped at him too and went pounding down the pavement with tears streaming down my face.

The next morning I asked my oncologist to feel the lymph node, and I saw her face assume the identical stricken look as had my husband's. Trying to comfort me, she commented on a small rash on the back of my neck, suggested it might be related, and said we could wait a week rather than rushing to a biopsy. Her cover of nonchalance was blown later that afternoon when my surgeon called me to say she had heard about my lymph node and to come and see her.

There is no right or wrong way to proceed in such a situation. If this node were cancerous, it would make no difference whether it was identified that day or several weeks later. I understood all too well the dire implications of a metastasis, and I could not bear to begin the trauma of facing such a diagnosis. I said I was not ready to deal with this and would call her in two weeks if the node was still there. I knew she was not happy with this response, but I did not change my mind. Other women might have opted to go immediately for a biopsy. Whether it was denial or fear or anger or just plain stubbornness, I could not do this. Instead I tried, with very limited success, to keep my fingers off the node and forced myself through the next days. A week later, the rash on the back of my neck was more pronounced, and this gave me hope that the node was a reaction to the rash. The worried looks from my husband and my doctor, however, suggested that it did not feel like a reactive lymph node to their practiced fingers. By the end of the second week, both the rash and the node were gone.

It was a horrendous experience, and it taught me several important lessons. First, it reminded me that I do not always behave with grace and courage. Second, I relearned the importance of knowing one's own style and needs. Whether you find it helpful to seek immediate investigation of a possible new problem or whether you opt to hide from it for a while is up to you. Obviously you cannot hide forever if the problem persists, but you do have a little time to keep the possibilities to yourself. Finally, it proved that sometimes there is indeed a happy ending. Having had breast cancer, it is tough to convince yourself that things can turn out well. They can and often they do.

Medical Follow-Up in Summary:

- Understand that you will be seeing your cancer doctors for a long time, if not for the rest of your life.
- Expect that these appointments will make you anxious. Many women find the week before a meeting with a doctor to be very difficult. If you do have tests such as blood tests or scans, waiting for the results is certain to be extremely stressful. Think about ways to make this period easier for yourself. Perhaps you can plan an evening with friends the night before your appointment or a special dinner the night after you have met with your doctor. Consider whether it makes you feel better or worse to take someone with you to your appointments and plan accordingly.
- Understand that the frequency of visits will diminish after the first two or three years.
- Try to stagger your appointments with your doctors. That is, if you are checking in with both your surgeon and your medical oncologist every six months, space the appointments so you see one of them every three months.
- Talk with your doctor(s) about what will help you feel well cared for and safe. For example, if you need reassurance about something, is it better to e-mail or to phone him? Do you need to again talk about your pathology

report or details of your treatment, or would you prefer to focus only on the here and now?

- Remember that at this stage the primary responsibility for the close monitoring of your health is shifting. Rather than relying on your doctors for your care, take responsibility for yourself.

- Most important, remind yourself that as long as you are feeling well, you are very likely to be fine!

6

Hormonal Therapies

Hormonal therapies are effective systemic treatments for breast cancer for women with estrogen-receptor-positive tumors. Like chemotherapy, they treat the whole body and are intended to kill any remaining cancer cells. The purpose of all hormonal therapies is to reduce or eliminate estrogen production, because estrogen stimulates the production of breast cancer cells—if those cells are estrogen-receptor positive. Women whose breast cancer is estrogen-receptor negative are not treated by hormonal therapies, because their cancer cells do not depend upon estrogen for their growth. The primary source of estrogen in premenopausal women is their ovaries. After menopause, whether natural or induced chemically or surgically, smaller amounts of estrogen are still produced by the adrenal glands.

Some women are treated with both chemotherapy and hormonal therapy, while others receive only hormonal therapy. If you are starting tamoxifen or an aromatase inhibitor after completing chemotherapy, it is likely that it will hardly feel like treatment. Taking a daily pill is a far different experience from receiving IV chemotherapy! Both tamoxifen and aromatase inhibitors share the same objective—reducing estrogen in your body—but they work in different ways. Tamoxifen blocks cancer cells' ability to take in and use estrogen, while the aromatase inhibitors reduce the amount of estrogen available in your body.

Treatments directed at changing the hormone environment in your body are very powerful and helpful therapies. They are also easy to take and cause few of the life-altering side effects that accompany most forms of chemotherapy. Tamoxifen (Nolvadex) is the most commonly prescribed hormonal therapy for women with estrogen-receptor-positive breast cancer. It was approved in the U.K. in 1973 and in the United States in 1977 for the treatment of advanced (metastatic) disease in postmenopausal women. This is a fairly standard way that new cancer treatments are used—first in the care of very ill patients. Then, if they prove to be helpful, they are evaluated in the care of people with earlier stages of cancer. By now, tamoxifen has been widely tested in the treatment of women with early breast cancer and found to be extremely helpful. Therefore, along with surgery and often radiation, it is commonly part of a woman's first, or adjuvant, treatment for breast cancer as well as continuing to be a valuable treatment for women who have metastatic breast cancer.

Some women, both pre- and postmenopausal, take tamoxifen for five years as their sole systemic treatment. Others first receive chemotherapy and then take tamoxifen for five years. This five-year duration has been shown to reduce the risk of a recurrence of a known breast cancer, to improve survival statistics, and to lower the risk of developing a second new breast cancer in the same or the other breast.

An analysis of women with both estrogen-receptor-positive and -negative breast cancers in the recent Tamoxifen Breast Cancer Prevention Trial, presented at the American Society of Clinical Oncology meeting in 2000, confirmed the value of this drug in the prevention of new breast cancers. Since women who have already had one breast cancer are at the top of the risk list for developing a new breast cancer, this confirmation is extremely important. If your breast cancer was diagnosed and treated some time ago and your doctor did not talk with you about tamoxifen, it is worth asking about its value for you now. The ways that drugs are used change over time, and it may be that it is now appropriate for you to consider this possibility.

Tamoxifen is also being prescribed for women who are at high risk for developing breast cancer because of genetic factors; this is discussed in detail in Chapter 15.

There is controversy about the use of tamoxifen for women whose breast cancer cells are estrogen-receptor negative. Some oncologists believe that it may also benefit them, if not in the treatment of their known breast cancer, then in reducing the risk of a second cancer. However, there have also been some studies suggesting that estrogen-receptor-negative women who take tamoxifen do not fare as well with their known cancer as women who do not take it. Since the data are unclear, your psychological well-being may be a factor in making this decision. This is another important conversation you may wish to have with your doctor.

Pat, a fifty-two-year-old elementary-school principal,

said, "I understand that I may not be helping myself and might even be hurting myself by taking tamoxifen. However, my doctor and I have talked a lot about this, and she is not concerned about the negative impact of tamoxifen in my case. Since I am so worried about a possible recurrence of my breast cancer, we both feel that taking tamoxifen is the right decision for me. I sleep better at night because I swallow that little pill right before I go to bed."

How does this little pill work? Breast cancer cells that are estrogen-receptor positive require estrogen to survive and multiply. In what is described as a "lock and key" arrangement, the cell must take in estrogen. Tamoxifen tricks any cancer cells—the "lock"—so that they perceive tamoxifen as the "key" and take it in, making them unable to take in estrogen. This results in the death of the cells.

Commonly described as an antiestrogen or an estrogen blocker, tamoxifen inhibits the growth of estrogen-receptor-positive (ER+) breast cancer cells while providing some of the benefits of estrogen to other parts of a woman's body; it helps maintain bone density and cardiac health in the same ways that estrogen would. For some women, tamoxifen also helps maintain some vaginal lubrication; for others, however, the converse is true.

For most of us, however, the most important benefit is the drug's anticancer effect. Tamoxifen reduces the risk of both local and distant recurrence of breast cancer between 30 and 45 percent. This means, for example, that if your risk of recurrence was estimated to be 20 percent, tamoxifen would reduce that 20 percent by 30 to 45 percent; your risk of recurrence would therefore be between 11 percent and 14 percent.

Tamoxifen is usually prescribed in a dose of 20 mg daily, taken either as a single 20-mg tablet or as two 10-mg tablets. For most women, the most difficult part of taking the drug is remembering to take it! If your doctor has told you to take one 10-mg tablet twice a day, this can be especially hard. It helps to set up a system. Some women keep the pill bottle next to their toothbrush to remind them to take the medicine twice daily. Others move the bottle from the right to the left side of the sink, or vice versa, each time. Some women buy a daily pill reminder box at the pharmacy and load it with two tablets for each day; this makes it easy to check a particular day's compartment. If you do forget to take a dose, do not assume that you should double up on the next one. Tamoxifen remains in your system for a long time; it has what is called a very long half-life. Your doctor may prefer that you skip that dose and then continue with the usual schedule.

The two serious potential complications of long-term tamoxifen therapy are an increased risk of endometrial cancer in the lining of the uterus and the development of blood clots, or thrombosis. If either of these rare complications were to happen to you, you would know it. Endometrial cancer causes vaginal bleeding, and blood clots cause pain and often swelling in the affected area. But the overwhelming health risk in your life is a recurrence of your breast cancer, and you will want to keep in mind the fact that your oncologist would not have prescribed tamoxifen if she felt that its risks outweighed its benefits.

There is some controversy regarding screening for endometrial cancer in women who are taking tamoxifen. It is helpful to remember that the risk is very small. An average woman's risk is approximately 3 per 1000, and tamoxifen increases that risk to 8 per 1000 women. Most endometrial cancers are highly curable by hysterectomy and give warning of their presence by bleeding. Most instances of spotting are harmless but are a signal to see your gynecologist.

If you find that you are quite anxious about the small risk of developing this cancer, you can talk with your doctor about annual transvaginal sonography or ultrasound. Although many oncologists have concluded that these are not necessary, others and some gynecologists prefer that their patients have this test each year. Since tamoxifen can cause the endometrial layer to thicken, the transvaginal ultrasound is often interpreted as abnormal. An abnormal result means an almost automatic recommendation of an endometrial biopsy—which then, in almost all instances, comes back normal. This sequence of events is anxiety-producing and usually serves no positive medical purpose. Again, since vaginal spotting or bleeding is the signal for any genuine problem, many doctors feel that it is perfectly safe and wise to omit these annual examinations.

If you or your doctor do feel that a transvaginal ultrasound is indicated, it is helpful to know what to expect. Transvaginal ultrasound is a painless and noninvasive screening that finds endometrial pathology. You are asked to disrobe from the waist down and assume the familiar gyn examination position. A sheet is draped over your knees and legs, and the technician hands you a wand that may be covered by a condom. You are asked to insert this into your vagina, and the technician then performs a standard ultrasound on your abdomen. If thickening or other abnormality of the uterine wall, or endometrium, is found, you will be advised to have an endometrial biopsy.

An endometrial biopsy, performed by a gynecologist, can be uncomfortable or painful. If you need to undergo this procedure, there are a few things that may help. The pain is quick and you can certainly manage it. You can also ask your doctor for a prescription for Ativan or Valium or another antianxiety medication when making the appointment. A small dose half an hour before the test will help relax you and is safe as long as you are not driving yourself home immediately afterward. You can also wear a Walkman and listen to music; it may be helpful to meditate; and practicing the relaxation response or deep breathing will also be of help.

Almost always, the endometrial-biopsy results come back normal, and this fact is the reason for the controversy about regular screening. Women taking tamoxifen should definitely continue with annual pelvic examinations and Pap tests and report any abnormal bleeding to their doctor. If an endometrial biopsy is indicated, in the unlikely event that cancer is found, it would be treated by hysterectomy.

The second possible serious consequence of long-term tamoxifen therapy is blood clots, or thrombosis. As rare as they are, blood clots are even less likely for younger, more active women. Clots tend to form in the leg veins and can become dangerous if they travel to the lung and block a blood vessel there; this is called a pulmonary embolism. The possibility of developing a blood clot while taking tamoxifen is approximately 8 in 1,000. Ask your doctor about the advisability of taking a single aspirin daily to reduce this risk even further. Aspirin is an anticoagulant, and a daily aspirin is known to be helpful in reducing other health risks; many oncologists feel that it is also prudent for their patients on tamoxifen. Blood-clot symptoms include redness, swelling, or discomfort in the legs, sudden chest pain, or shortness of breath. If any of these develops, call your doctor right away. While this very rare side effect is potentially dangerous, it does produce warning signals to seek help at once.

The most common side effect of tamoxifen is hot flashes. If they are severe, ask your doctor about medication that can reduce their number and intensity (see Chapter 4). Other possible side effects include weight gain, headaches, nausea, and mood swings. However, some studies have reported a similar number of such symptoms in women given a placebo; this makes it more difficult to be certain that such reactions are due to tamoxifen and not to other factors. Except for weight gain (and, yes, most women do gain between five and fifteen pounds), these side effects are likely to diminish or disappear over time. The most unpleasant ones, nausea and headaches, do not tend to last more than a few weeks and can be treated in the usual ways. Rare instances of disturbances in vision or irritation of the liver have been described in the medical literature.

Some women experience very painful leg cramps, especially at night. Drinking a glass of tonic—quinine water—before you go to bed may prevent them. It is also possible to take quinine in pill form; ask your doctor. Marilyn, a retired nurse, suggested turning around in bed so that your head is at the foot of the bed and your feet are at the head. Then bend your legs and push your feet flat, as hard as you can, against the headboard of the bed or the wall. Several women who have tried this exercise report that it helps—and one was astonished that her husband slept through the whole process!

A few women do experience side effects from tamoxifen that are sufficiently uncomfortable to warrant a change in therapy. Alice, a forty-year-old nurse, had a small and early breast cancer that was treated with a wide excision, radiation therapy, and tamoxifen. Starting a week after she began taking the drug, she had daily headaches. She consulted with her oncologist, who reassured her that they were rare and most certainly would disappear in a few weeks. They did not. She had headaches daily for a full year before she finally told her oncologist about them. She had kept them to herself because she desperately wanted to continue taking what she knew was a powerful anticancer treatment. When she finally spoke up, she was offered the choice of changing to another antiestrogen therapy or stopping hormone therapy altogether. After much deliberation, she decided that she was comfortable stopping the tamoxifen and not replacing it. Her headaches immediately ceased.

Nonetheless, many oncologists feel that the only advisable reasons for stopping tamoxifen are life-threatening side effects, such as endometrial cancer or thrombosis, or if taking the drug is sufficiently detrimental to the quality of life to outweigh the known benefits of the therapy. This is a decision that must be carefully made between doctor and patient.

Sometimes cost is a serious consideration. If your medical insurance does not have a prescription benefit, you probably are worried about the expense of tamoxifen.

There are a couple of helpful possibilities. As you probably know, most prescription drugs are significantly less expensive in Canada than they are in the United States. Ask your doctor about reliable sources, often through the Internet, of drugs in Canada. If your finances are even tighter, Astra-Zeneca, the manufacturer of tamoxifen, has a financial-assistance program that can sometimes provide the drug at no cost. Ask your doctor or social worker for assistance.

Studies to determine the optimal duration of tamoxifen therapy have found five years to be the recommended course. It provides more benefit than two years and, perhaps surprisingly to nonmedical people, the same benefit as ten years. There is also the rare possibility that at some point after five years of therapy, tamoxifen may begin to act like an estrogen rather than an estrogen blocker, and there is no way to identify those women in whom this change might happen. Should it occur, the drug presumably could "feed" any remaining cancer cells rather than prevent their growth.

Aromatase Inhibitors

Aromatase is an enzyme that produces estrogen in fat tissue. (Note that this is the reason that being overweight—having excess fat—is sometimes on the list of risk factors for breast cancer.) In postmenopausal women, most of the estrogen produced in the body obviously does not come from the ovaries; it is produced in the adrenal glands. Estrogen results from the conversion of a substance called a precursor steroid into estrogen with the assistance of the aromatase enzyme. Drugs that interfere with this natural process cause estrogen depletion and therefore starve estrogen-receptor-positive breast cancer cells of the hormone that is critical for their growth. Thus, aromatase inhibitors and ta-moxifen have the same desired result—the death of any remaining breast cancer cells—but achieve it through different biological mechanisms.

Aromatase inhibitors (including Arimidex, Femara, and Aromasin) form another category of hormonal therapy that has recently been introduced in the care of women with early-stage breast cancer. These drugs have been used for many years in the treatment of metastatic breast cancer, as well as in the treatment of the few women who have difficulty taking tamoxifen. What is a new and developing trend is their use *instead* of tamoxifen for some women receiving adjuvant treatment for early breast cancer.

Recently, a study comparing an aromatase inhibitor and tamoxifen in the initial treatment of women who developed metastatic breast cancer indicated that the response rates were somewhat higher with the aromatase inhibitor. This finding stimulated a clinical trial comparing tamoxifen to Arimidex, an aromatase inhibitor, in women with early breast cancer (a cancer in the breast without known metastases). The results of the trial indicated that the women who were taking Arimidex (anastrozole) experienced significantly fewer recurrences of breast cancer than did the women who were taking tamoxifen. Clinical trials are ongoing to compare the benefits of aromatase inhibitors to those of tamoxifen. Although this first study was certainly encouraging, it is premature to conclude that further data will uphold it. It is also not yet known if women taking Arimidex will have better survival rates.

The side effects of aromatase inhibitors are few. A small number of women have diarrhea, and there is also the possibility of increased osteoporosis. Aromatase inhibitors do not provide tamoxifen's positive benefits to bone density and cardiac functioning. There is some concern that women taking aromatase inhibitors are at higher risk for osteoporosis because of the very low or absent levels of estrogen in their bodies. Some oncologists recommend that their patients taking aromatase inhibitors have bone-density examinations every eighteen months to two years. Whether or not an aromatase inhibitor is right for you can only be decided after a thorough discussion with your oncologist.

It can be upsetting and confusing to hear about the value of other antiestrogen drugs. News reports are often misleading. There is so much ambiguity about breast cancer and its treatment that hearing that drug X may be more effective than tamoxifen can be worrisome. If you wonder about such reports and whether some other drug might be better for you, by all means talk with your doctor about it. Probably you will be reassured that tamoxifen, with its long and positive track record, is exactly the right choice. It may prove that recent and ongoing information about the value of aromatase inhibitors will gradually change the current standard of care. All these are decisions to be carefully made with your doctor who knows your particular situation best.

Scientists and physicians who are studying whether some other hormonal therapies may be even better than tamoxifen are also looking at whether any of them might be used in addition to tamoxifen. A large national study is now under way that offers estrogen-receptor-positive women who are completing five years of tamoxifen therapy the opportunity to participate in a clinical trial. This double-blind study compares the addition of five years of letrozole (Femara), an aromatase inhibitor, and a placebo. The question being explored is whether the addition of five years of an aromatase inhibitor will improve recurrence and survival rates. Femara has been used for some years, especially in Europe, in the treatment of metastatic breast cancer. It prevents the manufacture of estrogen anywhere in the body in postmenopausal women. As noted earlier in the discussion about tamoxifen, most cancer therapies are initially tested and used in individuals who have advanced disease. If the results are promising, they are then tested sooner in the course of an illness; this is now the situation with Femara. Since this study of giving women five years of Femara after five years of tamoxifen has just begun, it will be years before we know whether the additional hormonal treatment will lower the incidence of late recurrences and, therefore, improve the survival rates for women with breast cancer.

When the time comes to stop the tamoxifen, you can expect to feel much as you did when you completed your course of chemotherapy. It is very reassuring to know that you are taking a powerful means of fighting the cancer, so ending treatment can be frightening. Remind yourself that the protective actions of tamoxifen have been found to extend beyond the therapy; its beneficial effects are thought to continue for years thereafter. Remind yourself, too, that the risk of a recurrence of breast cancer diminishes with each passing year and that you are, at this point, more than five years past your diagnosis.

If any side effects of tamoxifen, particularly the hot

flashes, have persisted throughout the treatment, you can expect them to stop when you stop taking the drug. Many women have told me that their hot flashes literally stopped within a week or two. Unfortunately, any weight gain associated with tamoxifen does not vanish, and it is not likely to be any easier losing those extra pounds than it has been in the past.

There is one more very important point to be made about hormone therapy following chemotherapy. It is always surprising to me that some women are intensely anxious, even resistant, about beginning tamoxifen or an aromatase inhibitor after completing their chemotherapy. Of course they are sick of taking drugs, of feeling ill, of being a patient and dependent on medications. Of course they would prefer to be done with any more drugs and to return to their precancer and pre-so-many-medications lives. However, the anticancer effects of hormone therapy are so well documented and the side effects—especially as compared to chemotherapy—are so minimal that it seems it should be a simple decision. Whatever the risks of tamoxifen or another hormone, the possible gains are enormous. For many women, hormone therapy is potentially more beneficial than the chemotherapy that came first.

Five years can seem endlessly long. You have finally gotten through the months of surgery, radiation, and chemotherapy and are very eager to resume your real life. For better or worse, cancer is now part of that real life, and hormone therapy is a powerful weapon on your side. Believe me when I reassure you that, very soon, taking a daily pill will not seem to be a big deal. If you give it much thought at all, it will likely be relief that you are still doing something so important to fight the cancer. Balance the real and proven benefits of the drug against whatever your personal reservations may be. Do remind yourself that breast cancer can be a very powerful enemy and it is never wise to underestimate its strength and cleverness. Anything you can do to maximize the chances that you will stay well should be done!

7

Complementary Therapies

Many women who have breast cancer explore the possible use of complementary or alternative or unorthodox therapies at some point during their experience. As you finish treatment and move into recovery, thinking about these therapies can be especially appealing. No matter how reassuring your doctors are about your future health, it is natural to feel that you need to do everything possible to keep the cancer at bay. During your active treatment, you may not have had the energy or time to learn about complementary therapies. You may also have worried that some of them might interfere with your chemotherapy or radiation, and it is highly likely that your doctor agreed with this view. Now, however, these treatments are behind you, and it is up to you and your body to carry on. You may find it reassuring and empowering to expand your wellness routines to include changes in your lifestyle. This is a good time to consider what is out there and to decide what, if anything, you wish to pursue.

There are very passionate feelings on both sides about the value of complementary therapies. However, there are a few basic points to remember about the use of any complementary therapies. There is very little truly objective evidence proving that any complementary therapies are beneficial against cancer. Western medicine is data-based and relies on careful clinical trials and studies for its theories, knowledge, and recommendations. It is estimated that fewer than half of American physicians receive any information about complementary therapies during their training. Medical schools are slowly starting to address this gap, but it will be a very long time, if ever, before sufficient attention is paid to this area. Many doctors are critical of these therapies and professionally unwilling to accept as helpful any treatment that has not been examined by the models that define medical science. It is obvious that there is a real need for more-rigorous study of complementary therapies and publication of any data that are obtained.

Clinical trials—the basis of medical research and care in this country—have not been widely done to determine the benefit of these therapies. The National Institutes of Health (NIH) had a $92 million budget in 2001, up from a mere $2 million a decade earlier, to study complementary/alternative treatments. The focus of the NIH is broad and wide, including, for example, the study of ginkgo biloba to prevent Alzheimer's disease, yoga to help insomnia, acupuncture to help arthritis, and massage to treat lower-back pain.

There is now a Center for the Study of Complementary

Medicines at the National Cancer Institute (NCI), so more data-based information will become available in the years ahead. It will then be much easier to make thoughtful choices. In the meantime, the NCI maintains an excellent Web site with information that is reliable and helpful; see the "Resources" section.

As matters stand now, women are both on their own and exposed to an overwhelming amount of information and strong opinion about these therapies. Because there are limited data about the efficacy of these treatments, it is vital to learn about the possible risks as well as to assess the validity of the proclaimed benefits. It is obvious that some choices, such as Reiki, have no possible negative side effects. It is equally obvious that others, such as intensive vitamin programs or the use of multiple Chinese herbs, are less easy to evaluate and may bring some negative or even harmful consequences. Large doses of certain vitamins may be toxic and can even cause kidney or liver failure. No one knows exactly what is in those bunches of herbs or whether some of them could be bad for you. Just as it is untrue that all medical treatments will turn out to be helpful for any particular individual, it is untrue that because complementary therapies are "natural," they can do no harm. As general summation, treatments that are external (e.g., massage, Reiki) cannot hurt you, while treatments that you ingest or otherwise take into your body have the potential to harm you. Be careful.

It is very difficult to sort through all the information, opinions, and claims about the value of these different procedures, diets, and treatments. Indeed, it is difficult even to know what to call them. Most of us are comfortable with the term *complementary therapies* to describe those that are used in addition to traditional Western medicine. This can mean adding acupuncture or Reiki or diet or any of a myriad of other possible therapies to the standard treatments of surgery, radiation, and hormonal or chemotherapy. *Alternative treatments,* strictly defined, are those that are used *instead* of conventional Western medicine. As with any illness, some women with breast cancer do opt for alternative or unconventional treatment only. I very much hope that this has not been your decision. I firmly believe in the power and value of both conventional Western medicine and, for some women, the additional value of complementary care.

A seminal article on the use of unconventional medicine in the United States was written by David Eisenberg, M.D., and his colleagues in 1993 (*unconventional* is the term that was used in this study). They conducted a national survey to study the prevalence, costs, and patterns of use of these therapies. Asking respondents about both their medical problems and their use of unconventional therapies, they found that one in three respondents (34 percent) had used at least one unorthodox therapy in the previous year, and that a third of these people had met with a practitioner for the treatment. Especially surprising and very worrisome was the additional finding that 72 percent of people who had used unconventional therapies had not told their medical doctors that they had done so.*

It is my guess that Eisenberg's figure of 34 percent is low when compared to the use of complementary therapies

*Eisenberg et al., "Unconventional Medicine in the United States," *New England Journal of Medicine,* 328:246–252, January 28, 1993.

by cancer patients. Thinking of women with breast cancer, it is certainly possible that those who choose to come to my support groups or to individual psychotherapy sessions are the same ones who are interested in exploring complementary therapies. My best estimate is that close to 90 percent of the women whom I meet at least consider the use of one of these therapies. Many others, of course, go through breast cancer without this kind of extra psychosocial support and do not use nontraditional therapies.

The list of complementary therapies that are used by women with breast cancer is long. I have known women who tried nutritional therapies, Reiki, therapeutic touch, exercise programs, herbs, Ayurvedic therapy, massage, meditation, hypnosis, chiropractic treatments, acupuncture, nutritional supplements, Essiac tea, shark or bovine cartilage, prayer, support groups, psychotherapy, dance or music or art therapy, visualization, vitamins, yoga, minerals, naturopathy, biofeedback, and trips to special clinics or practitioners in other countries. Clearly no one person could possibly do or want to do all of these things; some are very controversial while others are almost mainline. The point is that there are many, many complementary therapies available, each with its proponents and critics. It can be daunting to try to figure out which are legitimate and might make a real contribution to your physical or emotional health.

There are several moments in the continuum of breast cancer care when a woman is most likely to think about complementary therapies. The first is around the time of diagnosis. During those initial days and weeks, most women are desperate to find and do anything that might help them. Some decide to use a combination of standard medical care and complementary therapies; others decide to delay the other therapies until their radiation or chemotherapy is completed. Many doctors are wary of adverse interactions between these treatments and chemotherapy or radiation. Moreover, there is biochemical evidence that certain alternative therapies can neutralize radiation or chemotherapy, so it is prudent to wait until these treatments are completed. Doctors are less likely to be critical about external treatments and may even encourage acupuncture, stress-reduction courses, or exercise. Those women who do choose to use nontraditional treatments in parallel with their standard care are *strongly* urged to be certain that their doctors, both their medical and their complementary providers, are aware of everything they are doing.

The second point at which complementary therapies become a strong interest is after the completion of standard treatment. As we have discussed, most women feel quite anxious about ending active anticancer therapy, and a good way to feel more empowered and in control is to learn about other ways to help yourself. It can be easier to move forward with the addition of therapeutic massage or diet supplements than without any active attempt (other than possibly going on tamoxifen or other hormone therapy) to continue fighting the cancer. Many women are aware of the current limits of conventional breast cancer treatments and want to do anything that might help keep them well.

Finally, women who are living with metastatic disease are obviously motivated to add any potentially helpful treatment to their regimens. When cure is no longer the focus, and a woman and her doctor are treating her cancer as a chronic illness and trying to maximize both quality and length of life, complementary therapies may be especially helpful.

Once more, it is essential to repeat the point that *all* your caregivers must know about everything that you are doing. Because there is a split between conventional and complementary therapies, and misunderstanding or lack of understanding on both sides, it can seem difficult to be fully honest with them all. You may be apprehensive that your medical oncologist or your herbalist will be critical of the other's care. But even if this happens, it is absolutely vital that you share the whole truth with them. Your choices remain your choices, but if there are strong reasons to reconsider what you are doing, it is essential that you hear them. You need to know all you can if you are to care for yourself in the ways that are best for your physical and emotional health.

If you do choose to pursue complementary therapy, select practitioners with the same care that guided you in finding your doctors. As you did then, ask other women for recommendations, call the relevant professional associations, and check with your state licensing board to be sure that an individual is properly licensed. Ask an acupuncturist or nutritionist or any other clinician about his or her experience in caring for people who have had cancer. It does not especially matter whether they have treated women who have had breast cancer as opposed to having cared for cancer patients in general. Ask what their results have been and what they feel is most helpful to their clients. Ask what problems they hope to address and how their methods will work. Check their background and references. Ask about cost and about payment possibilities. Although a few medical-insurance plans will pay for certain kinds of complementary therapies (acupuncture, stress-reduction programs, or chiropractic services are the likeliest), you will have to pay out of pocket for most.

It is also important to beware of quacks! If something sounds too good to be true, it probably is. If claims seem exaggerated, or the costs seem very high, or the practitioner is unwilling to share information with your medical doctors, look elsewhere. There really are people out there preying on the fear and urgency of cancer patients.

Most women who are interested in complementary therapies when their active medical treatment is completed are hoping to boost their immune systems, enhance their overall sense of well-being, and destroy any cancer cells that might be left in their bodies. There is, however, no firm proof that the immune system can be altered to protect against cancer or to destroy cancer cells, and it is difficult, if not impossible, to ever really know whether any of these treatments can help you meet these goals. You can, however, evaluate their contribution to your sense of your health and of yourself as you move into the future. As long as something makes you feel better and is doing no harm, it is doing you good!

I have worked with women who have used many kinds of complementary therapies and who have believed that their use has been valuable. Many who are undergoing chemotherapy find that acupuncture reduces nausea and that Reiki improves their energy level. After treatment ends, it can be harder to evaluate the contribution of these therapies since, blessedly, you are starting to feel better anyway. Their value at this time is more in their impact on your overall sense of good health and optimism.

In China, in India, in Native American culture, in Africa, and in many other parts of the world, herbal medicine has a very long and distinguished history. It is thought to be as beneficial as more-modern Western medicine, and the two are frequently prescribed in tandem. Approximately 25 percent of all prescription drugs are derived, either directly or through synthesis in the laboratory, from the natural world. Remember that the term *natural* really means this: that the described substance was grown, not synthesized in a laboratory. It is not a guarantee of effectiveness or even safety; lots of poisons are natural substances. *Natural* has become a popular advertising term and is often misleading in its use. Describing something as natural is saying nothing at all about its intrinsic value.

The World Health Organization notes that most of these drugs are used by Western medicine in ways that parallel their traditional use. Eastern medicine views health as a balance between physiological and psychological factors, and cancer is seen as a result of a poorly functioning immune system. Therefore, combinations of herbs, usually eight to ten, are suggested to restore balance in an individual's system. Herbs can be taken either in pill form or boiled in a tea. Whether any of these therapies actually fight the cancer directly or whether they simply minimize treatment side effects and enhance overall well-being is unknown. In the setting of illness, however, feeling stronger may make it possible to accept difficult treatment, and that treatment can indeed prolong life.

Much of the concern and controversy about complementary therapies is about the value and use of herbal medicine. Since Western medicine and science have not yet studied most of these herbs and since it is impossible to know exactly what is in each one and how each may affect the body, most physicians' attitudes toward them range from skeptical to critical. A good example is the frequent use of herbs for the treatment of hot flashes. As has been noted earlier, hot flashes result from the loss of estrogen, and hormone-replacement therapy (HRT) cannot be used by women who have had breast cancer. (Moreover, recent studies of HRT have suggested that its value for any woman is questionable, and it is likely that more and more attention will be focused on alternatives.) There are a number of herbs and herbal preparations that can help to reduce hot flashes, but many contain plant estrogens (phytoestrogens) and so cannot be assumed to be safe for a woman who has had breast cancer. They are effective for hot flashes because they act like estrogen in the body. Herbs may seem natural and therefore harmless; remember that they *can* cause harm. The bottom line is that it is essential to know as much as possible about any herbal treatments that you are considering and to speak with your doctors about their use.

Acupuncture, another ancient form of Chinese medicine, has been better accepted by the mainstream culture; acupuncturists are even sometimes on staff at hospitals and cancer centers. An acupuncturist inserts needles (make sure they are disposable!) in any of four hundred or more specific points, along connecting lines called meridians, in the body. Benefits can include reduction in nausea, hot flashes, pain, anxiety, and depression. Believers also say that acupuncture can improve immune-system function, though there is no firm proof of this claim. Many acupuncture practitioners are also physicians, trained in the United States as well as in Asia. Women give mixed reports on whether acupuncture is uncomfortable. Some claim to feel nothing, others to feel mild to moderate discomfort when the needles are inserted.

There are a number of hands-on therapies that seem a natural continuation of the healing tradition. The laying on of hands has been recognized as therapeutic throughout human history. Massage, Reiki and Shiatsu, and therapeutic touch are examples of treatments that are safe and are very likely to feel good.

Nutrition and various nutritional therapies are the subject of as much controversy as the use of herbs. Bookstores and libraries are lined with books purporting to outline diets that will prevent or cure all manner of human illness and misery. There is even a so-called "breast cancer prevention diet"! It is prudent to be skeptical of any of these diets' claims, as are most physicians.

Whatever your inclinations, you will find that there are books or articles to support them. Most nutritionists who work in health-care settings believe in the value of a balanced diet and preach the importance of moderation in all things. There are well-known recommendations to eat at least five servings of fruit or vegetables daily and to reduce your intake of saturated fats. There are multiple variations of food pyramids, suggestions of how to balance grains, proteins, and fat, and opinions about the value of every part of a diet. It can seem that a new study is released every month that describes a different food or beverage as a culprit in causing cancer. It then often happens that subsequent studies debunk the earlier theory.

It is believed that approximately one-third of all cancers are in part the result of diet. Most of us know that the rate of breast cancer is lower in Japan and in China than in the Western world, but that the incidence rises when Japanese and Chinese women live in this country or in western Europe. Some scientists even suggest that the periods of greatest influence and therefore dietary risk are the times in life of rapid hormonal and body growth. This means that what your mother ate when she was pregnant with you or what you ate during adolescence may have been the most important. If this turns out to be true, making diet changes now will obviously have less impact on your health. Questions of the contribution of diet and other environmental or lifestyle factors to cancer are extremely complicated. The bottom line is that no one now really knows, or can prove, the influence of diet on the development or progression of breast cancer.

Clearly it behooves us all to use common sense in choosing what we eat. It also is sensible to question any claims that various foods, food products, and diets have an impact on the risk of cancer or its progression. Ask for the proof. It probably won't hurt you to eat a handful of nuts or a cup of carrot juice or a tablespoon of flaxseed daily. On the other hand, it *could* hurt you to avoid dairy products completely (you need that calcium!) or eat very large amounts of soy (remember that soy is a plant estrogen and may be dangerous if you have an estrogen-receptor-positive breast cancer) or take nutritional or diet or weight-reduction products.

Having breast cancer has taught us to value and enjoy our lives. Food is a major source of pleasure for many of us. We like to read about it, think about it, shop for it, cook it, and eat it. It would be a great pity to give up foods we love without solid evidence that they are harmful. I wish there were specific studies to quote or articles to recommend to you about what you eat. It would be reassuring to think that we could reduce our risk of recurrence through diet; it would give us some control. But there is no evidence to support this, so it all boils down to your deciding what makes you feel you are doing all you can to maintain good health.

After breast cancer you almost certainly are feeling differently about your body than you were before. To a greater or lesser degree, we are less trusting of our physical selves, more vulnerable to assaults from all sides, and feeling much less in control. Our culture tries to teach us that if we do everything right (diet, exercise, stress management, personal relationships, et al.), we will be rewarded with good health and long-lasting youth. We have learned that this is not true and that many of the major elements in life, including serious health problems, are largely beyond our control. Yes, there are known diet and exercise strategies to fight heart disease or to better control diabetes, but no one knows with certainty what causes cancer, no one knows with certainty why some cancers are apparently cured by appropriate treatment and why others return.

I believe that the intense interest and motivation many of us have to explore and use complementary therapies comes from this puzzle. We so want to believe that we can do *something* to keep ourselves healthy and prevent the cancer from recurring. Certainly, significant modifications to our diets or lifestyles can have positive impact on our overall health. We know that we are better off living with less stress, more exercise, and healthy diets but come to realize that an imperfect world and the realities of our lives and our health make any guarantees impossible. We are likely to be more skeptical of claims of promised health than are our friends who have not had cancer. This realization can help us to explore, consider, and perhaps adopt strategies that we believe may help us, as long as they are not dangerous. Whether any enhanced sense of well-being that results is actually due to a placebo effect is less important than the reality that when we sense we are more in control, we generally feel stronger.

8

Concerns of Husbands and Partners

Your husband or partner is exhausted and worried, too. He has lived with you through a very stressful period. Over the years I have worked with several women not only throughout their breast cancer experience but later, during their husbands' own cancer diagnosis and treatment. They have all said that, much to their surprise, it was easier in many ways to be the ill spouse. It has consistently been my experience that most husbands and partners rise to the immediate crisis and are as supportive and helpful to their wives as they can possibly be through the months of diagnosis and treatment. It has also consistently been my experience that the stresses and tensions are real and that very few couples navigate these difficult months without some problems. For most couples, time and your gradual recovery bring resolution of the strains. It is important to maintain faith in your relationship and in each other and to allow for some less-than-perfect moments. As is always the case, communication is key, and you will both need to keep talking to each other about your feelings and experiences.

You may have been initially worried that he would find you less desirable or even love you less as your body was changed, but you have made the necessary beginning adaptations together. A full discussion of sexuality and intimate concerns follows in Chapter 9, but it is probable that your intimate life together has suffered and that you will both need to find your way back to a mutually satisfying sex life.

Never underestimate the impact of your illness on your husband or partner. Like you, he is terrified about the future, afraid that the cancer may come back. His perspective differs from yours. You are scared and sad that your life may be shortened and that you may not live to experience many of life's joys. He is not only afraid that he will lose you, his beloved and his life partner, he is also anxious about how he would manage. Especially if you have young children, he worries about how he could care for them while continuing to work and have any kind of personal life. It is likely that he cannot express these fears to you, but you can be certain that he is thinking about them and is frightened and sad.

He has been dealing with other strong feelings as well. He may be angry that this has happened to you, to him, and to your family. Just as you felt that cancer was a most unwelcome intruder and a betrayal by your body, so did he. You were forced to put aside your life for these months. So was he. As you felt that you lost yourself, he felt that he lost his wife. Just as you sometimes barely recognized yourself, he sometimes barely recognized you.

Libby said: "My husband was my rock, always there for me, every step of the way. He does not talk about my cancer, never tells me that 'you are going to be fine,' but there is a quiet strength that helps to sustain me in my times of terror. I know he worries about me. But he doesn't talk about it. I suppose that is because he doesn't want to add fuel to the fire. I talk about it constantly and worry about every new ache or pain. Sometimes his silence makes me angry. I want him to tell me, 'You are going to be fine.' I want *someone* to tell me that I am going to be fine!"

Most husbands usually feel that part of their role is to protect their beloved, and your cancer has tested his capacity to do so. You have both been forced to acknowledge how much is out of your control and that some demons cannot be exorcised. Together you have been in the maelstrom, and together you have been tossed and buffeted. During the months of treatment, the focus was on your schedule and your needs. Your husband or partner is now eager to regain some balance in his own life, but you may feel that this shift in attention is happening all too quickly. While you continue to struggle with your intense feelings and your slow physical recovery, he may be acting as though life is back to normal. It is very important for the two of you to speak frequently and honestly about your needs and your feelings. One change, perhaps not so welcome, must come from you: It is both appropriate and fair that his voice now be heard equally and his wishes equally respected. You will need to renegotiate the balance in your relationship; you no longer have automatic claim to your view. Now that the active treatments are over, living your lives together must begin for you both.

As you slowly begin to heal, you need to make time for him again. It was not possible for you to expend psychic energy worrying about him during the acute crisis of your cancer. It is time now to remind yourself that you and he have a partnership and that you need to care for him and his needs just as he needs to continue to care for you and yours.

Even if your husband usually has good psychological insight and the capacity to talk about his feelings, your cancer has been a wholly different experience. How could he tell you how angry he is about your missing breast or how hard it was to see you feeling ill and weak? How could he tell you how scared and sad he was without feeling that he was burdening you? How could he tell you that he lay awake many nights wondering how he could possibly manage to raise your children alone? Many men share their feelings and vulnerability only with their wives, so if he found himself unable to speak of this to you, what could he do? Whom else could he tell about his anger or his fear of losing you; how could he acknowledge his sense of failure and impotence because he could not shelter you from this crisis? If you don't know the answers to these questions, ask him. The answers may or may not surprise you, but the conversation will be a step toward taking more-balanced care of each other.

At the right moment, ask him how this time has been for him. Tell him that you know he must be feeling angry or frightened or sad. If you can muster the courage, you might even say that you know he must sometimes think about what life would be like without you and how overwhelming that thought must be. You may not be able to talk with him in this way until you are feeling strong and well, and if you need to wait until you are sturdier and can bear his pain, that's fine. But have this conversation someday.

Many couples find that sessions with a counselor or therapist, especially one who is sophisticated about cancer and its treatment, are very helpful in this transition period. If you are struggling with marital problems or simply feeling that you have not been able to process cancer together, as a couple, it is worth considering this option. All marriages have issues and tensions, and those that existed between you before your breast cancer are still there. If you managed to put them aside during the months of treatment, they will resurface now and they may be more troubling than they were in the past.

Meg and Steven came to my office approximately six months after she completed chemotherapy. They had been married for twenty-two years, had two daughters, and had always believed they had a good relationship and a solid marriage. But as she regained her physical strength, Meg was surprised to recognize how angry she was with him and how puzzling these feelings were. In the course of our talking together over a period of about three months, she began to express her worry that they had grown apart and that he no longer loved her. Throughout her treatment he had been helpful and supportive in many practical ways but had withdrawn from her emotionally and sexually. Steven explained that she had always seemed to be feeling exhausted or sick and that he had been, and still was, afraid he would hurt her if they resumed their intimacy. He also began to understand his fear of the intense feelings that a sexual connection can create. These sessions were an opportunity for both to talk about how frightened they were about Meg's future health and to gradually understand that, by withdrawing from each other, they were trying to minimize the pain of a possible loss. Expressing these feelings brought them a shared sense of relief and a rapid improvement in their relationship.

Unfortunately, some husbands or partners are unable to handle the cancer, and I have known a few who left the relationship shortly after diagnosis. One woman's husband drove her home from the hospital following her surgery, put down her suitcase, and then said, "I can't do this." He left and never came back. Another stayed through his wife's course of chemotherapy, frequently making disparaging remarks about her bald head or absent libido, and moved out the day after her final radiation treatment.

Nor is it always the husband who cannot cope; sometimes the wife feels that she cannot continue a bad or shaky marriage. Recovering from cancer includes reflecting on all your important relationships, and life may seem too short to spend in an unhappy marriage. Some women who have been contemplating divorce but planning to wait until their children were older may decide that there is no longer time to wait. Others decide that their life is too precious to spend with a man who is alcoholic or emotionally abusive or simply distant. Some women want more from a relationship than their husband is able to give, and decide that it is worth the risk of leaving in the hope of eventually finding a more fulfilling partner.

If this is your experience, whether or not you are the instigator of a separation or divorce, you will now be contending with many problems beyond the usual ones of recovery. If you are in control of the decision or the timetable, I do suggest that it will be wise to wait until you can wait no longer. If possible, try not to take on this crisis now. If you can, give yourself at least a year to recover from your cancer.

Work at sustaining the normal rhythms of your own and your children's lives. It may be that as the months pass, you and your husband will find better ways to communicate and be together and may opt not to go ahead with a separation. You can use this time to do everything possible to muster all available resources and supports and to think about the shape of your new life. You can consult with a financial planner and an attorney. You will have time to consider your living arrangements and whether you would need to move, and you can talk with friends who have been through a divorce and listen to their experience and their wisdom. Slow and careful consideration of this vitally important decision will be a great help, whether in the end you decide to stay or to go. Take your time and keep reminding yourself that the most important goal right now is the gradual recovery of your own physical and emotional equilibrium.

Midway through my own course of chemotherapy, my husband and I spent a weekend away together in an attempt to enjoy each other and to take a brief respite from the rigors of treatment. While wandering through a gallery, we spotted an etching that seemed a perfect metaphor for our experience. He later called the gallery, spoke with the artist, and purchased the picture, and he gave it to me—a surprise and a delight—on the final day of my chemotherapy. It is two trees, one larger than the other, blowing in a gale. Their branches and leaves are twisted and their trunks are struggling to stay upright. The trees take up only the top third of the paper; the remainder is their roots—deep and intertwined, and filled with life as they hold strong. Below the surface is another world, bursting with energy and solace and meaning.

We have a different relationship and a different life to-gether than we would have had if I had not had cancer. Is it worse? Definitely not, as long as I stay well. Is it better? I'm not sure. I miss the ease and belief in unending happiness that we had before cancer. We used to laugh more. We have been personally reminded about vulnerability and limits and time and death. Over time, these lessons have become the patina of our relationship. Just like old silver, the shine is mellow and marred yet even more precious.

The reclaiming of life—for you, for him, and for you as a pair—will be slow and almost certainly not a smooth duet. Over and over I hear from recovering women that once past the cancer crisis, their husbands seem to behave as though life were back to normal. This is, of course, what your husband, like all who love you, wants to believe. Even when he is terrified and saddened by the uncertainty of the future, he is sometimes able to step out of cancer. When he is at work or on the golf course or playing with your chil-dren or grandchildren, he is probably not thinking cancer. You do not have that luxury nor that ability. At least for as long as your physical healing is incomplete and your face in the mirror looks unfamiliar, you will be holding court with the presence of your disease. Expect sometimes to be frus-trated or furious with his apparent nonchalance; try to re-member that he does not and cannot live inside your changed body and mind.

Leanne was treated for a very high-risk breast cancer ten years ago. She has stayed well but feels that her illness and treatment have irrevocably changed her marriage. She describes it as "just different." She believes that the impact of her cancer is a daily presence in her relationship with her husband. Part of it has been her loss of libido and their diminished sexual relationship. (This common reaction is fully discussed in Chapter 9.) But most of it, she says is because "he has no idea what I have been through. We are talking across two worlds." She has completely changed the way she thought about financially preparing for their future. Since she is the major breadwinner in their family, she feels increased pressure to earn and invest money to protect her children's future. She no longer feels that she has twenty years in which to build a sound financial plan. At the same time, it seems less urgent to plan for her own retirement and often more important to spend money now for trips or for things that she wants. There are still many days when "all of my emotions come flooding back" and, on those days, she feels especially and painfully distant from her husband.

There are, unfortunately, many women who sense that their marriages have been changed and sometimes damaged by their illness. A few strategies may help in preventing this outcome. Keeping the lines of communication open, expressing your feelings and fears even if he does not seem to understand, insisting that you listen to each other and honor each other's thoughts—all these will help. If at all possible, it would be an excellent idea for the two of you to get away alone together, ideally several months after the end of your treatment. As eager as you may be to mark its end and begin your post-cancer life, you will not be feeling strong enough or as eager to sample the pleasures of travel as you will be some weeks later. Your budget and other responsibilities will dictate whether this will be a single night in a nearby hotel, a few days at a resort, or a more major trip to a distant place. Where you go matters less than the time you carve out to be together. Just as a honeymoon marks an important transition in a relationship, this trip can signify the commitment to your new life. My husband and I followed this advice and spent a week away together a few months after my chemotherapy ended. As we arrived at our destination, a brief rainstorm ended and a vivid rainbow arched through the sky. There could have been no better metaphor.

It is also important to find ways, as a couple, to mark the cancer anniversary. It is obvious that you and your relationship were changed forever by cancer. It is likely that your husband or partner will find reasons to mark this anniversary obscure. He may well think that he would prefer to put it all behind as quickly as possible and never remember the date. Anniversary reactions are powerful. Even if you choose to ignore the date and even if you do "forget" it, it is very likely that you will find yourself filled with intense feeling each year as the day arrives. My opinion is that you do better to mark it. Reminding yourself and each other annually that this happened to you, that you have come through together, and that another year has passed will likely become even more important as time goes on. Each year of good health is a blessing to be acknowledged.

Some people honor the day of diagnosis, others the day of surgery or the final day of treatment. The specific date is far less important than taking time, together, to remember and note it. This is not likely to feel celebratory—not even when you are five or ten years past your illness. But on that day, you and your relationship were changed forever. In some ways this is as significant an event as your marriage or the birth of your children. Remember it and create a ritual to share.

Lesbian Couples

The stresses and issues for lesbian couples are both the same as for any other pair and different. At the beginning, many lesbian women feel especially well-supported by their partners. After all, another woman certainly understands what it feels like to have your breast changed or surgically removed, to lose your hair, to feel less womanly. Since women are generally more fluent than men in the language of emotional responsiveness, lesbian partners may be better able to express and talk about their feelings. It is generally assumed that two women will have a more nurturing relationship than will a man and a woman, but it can be dangerous to make broad generalizations about people and relationships. A lesbian partner may or may not have been any more consistently supportive than a husband.

The practicalities of living during breast cancer treatment are often easier for women. Both partners are likely to be competent with domestic responsibilities; I have never heard tales of lesbian partners being unable to cook or do laundry or make a child's lunch, unlike what is often said of husbands. Although a partner will have had to assume more of such responsibilities and of the emotional needs of the ill woman, overall she may not have been as stressed and exhausted by these demands, simply because they were familiar to her. It is slightly easier to do more when the tasks are already part of your routine.

I have been particularly impressed by the response of

the lesbian community in general during times of stress with breast cancer. This may be true for other situations as well, but the outpouring of help and affection is a regular occurrence following a breast cancer diagnosis. Since data indicate that the incidence of breast cancer is somewhat higher among lesbian than among straight women, this community has had to think all too often of its responsibility and responsiveness to one another. Several women have told me that their friends organized themselves so that every single night during the months of treatment, someone came to their home, cooked and served dinner, cleaned up, and then went home. While the downside for this kind of community support may be a loss of privacy and perhaps some sense for the well partner that she isn't thought to be fully up to the job, most of us would definitely feel that the benefit outweighs the cost!

One significant issue for lesbian couples, and to a lesser extent for unmarried heterosexual couples, can be the attitudes of health-care providers. One of my patients was initially diagnosed with breast cancer at another Boston hospital but came to Beth Israel Deaconess for her care. She recalled that her first surgeon, who performed her breast biopsy and made the diagnosis, did not invite her partner into the examination room and refused to treat her as the primary person in the patient's life. In contrast, her surgeon at Beth Israel Deaconess, upon being told that her partner had first felt the breast lump, turned to her and said, "Good call! You may have saved her life." Another woman reported that her surgeon, after telling her that she needed bilateral mastectomies, said, "You probably always wanted the flat-chested look." For a variety of complicated reasons, she did not change surgeons at that time, but she did decide to find another doctor once her treatments were completed.

It is extremely important, in terms of feeling secure and well cared for by your doctors, that they are fully accepting of a same-sex partnership. It is equally important to the health of that partnership that you both feel respected and included in the medical care. Since I hear from my lesbian patients that "it is mostly otherwise," meaning that all too many health-care providers do not treat their partners as they would a male partner or a husband, I urge you to pay careful attention to this and to feel free to change doctors if this acceptance is not forthcoming.

Lesbian partners may also have experienced difficulty in their work or larger worlds. Not everyone lives or works in an environment that is accepting of same-sex relationships. If your partner cannot tell her boss or coworkers about your cancer, she will certainly feel more alone and isolated, and she will not be offered the kind of flexibility that benefits many husbands as they care for their wives. This difficult situation is likely to impose an additional stress within the relationship. Again, recognizing the tension and talking together about it as you go forward with your lives will be helpful.

Many partners find it most useful to talk with other partners who have experienced similar problems. A woman who has helped her partner through breast cancer can be an ideal confidante for these discussions. Just like husbands, partners are saddened and frightened by what you have been through and what may lie ahead. The same fears of losing you, of having to create a new life, perhaps of having to raise children alone are there. You yourself may have the same worries that a wife would regarding her future and that of your children. Would your partner have the same patience with them that you do? Would she read to them each night or understand their dreams? Would she do what you would do and give what you would give?

In summary, there are more similarities than differences in all committed relationships. The fact of your breast cancer may feel like a third party intruding into your relationship for a very long time. You will both be deeply affected by it and your relationship will be different than what it would have been without cancer. Your solo life will not be the same, nor will your life as a couple. In both instances, the goal is to find and establish a new rhythm and together to craft it to reflect and honor what you now know to be most important and valuable.

9

Sexuality

Sex is one way that we say, "I'm alive!" The sensations, the intimacy, the closeness and sense of healthy well-being that it creates is unique. It is probable that your sex life will be less gymnastic or intense for a while, but making love may matter even more. Now that you and your partner have both been painfully forced to recognize your mortality and vulnerability, coming together intimately seems even more precious. The act that creates life also celebrates and savors it.

When you were first diagnosed with breast cancer and during the months of your active treatment, it is probable that sexuality was not a primary concern; indeed, passionate sex may have been one of the very last things of interest to you. Certainly physical and emotional intimacy with your partner was important during those months, but it is likely that you also found ways of loving and supporting each other that were not sexual. Being close, being held, feeling secure and safe in each other's arms were more necessary than passion. Now that your treatment is over, however, sex probably will become important again.

Nonetheless, when the acute crisis has passed and you are trying to reclaim your life, you may well find that you have a diminished libido and less enjoyment in sex. If you are now in menopause, some of this is the result of your hormonal changes—specifically the loss of estrogen and testosterone, both of which play a part in sexual response. Even if you are still menstruating, your body feels different and probably responds less intensely than it used to. Whatever your hormones are or are not doing, your mind has been elsewhere over the past months. This can seem yet another loss, one more way that breast cancer has negatively changed your life. As one of my patients said when I asked her about this part of her marriage: "What sexuality?" Any preexisting problems with sexuality or with your relationship in general have probably been exacerbated by your cancer and by its treatment. Some of this may be directly related to physical and hormonal changes from your treatment, and some may have its roots in the history of your relationship and the impact of cancer on it.

Even without breast cancer, many women begin to experience problems with their sexuality as they age. Although breast cancer certainly targets far too many young women, its incidence is higher in older women. That is, the combination of normal aging and the aftereffects of breast cancer treatment combine to cause sexual difficulties for many postmenopausal women. Many women have difficulty with arousal and orgasm and may feel much less interested in sex in general. Some even experience pain with intercourse. And, of course, the partners of older women are likely to be older themselves and perhaps experiencing their own challenges with sexual performance. All of these problems may be greater for women following breast cancer treatment.

If you do perceive that you are having sexual problems, whom do you talk to about them? You yourself may not be comfortable with this topic, and most oncologists do not talk about sex with their patients before, during, or after treatment. From the doctor's perspective, sexual issues are not at the top of the list of medical concerns. She is more worried about delivering the right treatment, sustaining you through it, and being vigilant for signs or symptoms of further trouble in the future. Moreover, the fact that someone is medically trained does not guarantee that he or she will be comfortable talking about sex. The same hang-ups and embarrassments that affect nonmedical people affect doctors, too. In addition, their reticence may derive from their own lack of knowledge about normal sexual response as well as about possible remedies for such problems in women following breast cancer.

It is most important that you be able to talk with your partner. Some couples find it easy to talk about sex and others don't. If you find it uncomfortable, consider writing a short note about your concerns. Allowing the written words to begin the dialogue may make conversation easier.

People have varying sexual needs, and it is possible that you are satisfied with your current level of response and activity. Most women have less sex during their cancer treatments and for a time—sometimes for a long time—

afterward. But if you're feeling that your partner is holding back, ask why. It may be that he is worried about physically hurting you and needs reassurance that your body is no longer so tender. As long as both of you can talk about it and are content with similar sexual patterns, whether that means once a day or twice a year, there is no problem.

It can be especially ironic and problematic if your own cancer treatment results in sexual changes that coincide with changes in your partner. Part of normal aging for men is a diminishment of their testosterone level and a lessened libido and capacity to achieve an erection. The seemingly boundless sexual vigor of youth is gone in most middle-aged and older men. It is difficult for you to experience and acknowledge the changes in your body and your sexuality. It is probably even harder for your partner to accept this in himself. Even more than women, most men are identified with and proud of their sexual prowess and appetites. The combination of normal aging, some difficulty achieving erection or orgasm on demand, and concern about hurting you can be damaging to your partner's sexual performance. Since he is likely to be ashamed and embarrassed about this, it is hard for him to talk about it. Performance anxiety often predicts difficulty with performance; the more concerned he is about whether he can have a lasting erection, the less likely it is that he will be able to do so. A couple of sexual experiences that don't go well and end in frustration for you both will make future intimacy harder.

Caitlin, a fifty-year-old woman in a very happy second marriage, had this very problem. "John is five years older than I am and was already occasionally having troubles with erections. Since my treatment and menopause, I have terrible dryness and not much interest. John got a prescription for Viagra, and I think it has made things even worse."

Although Viagra acted as advertised and enabled him to have and sustain an erection, the drug also gave him headaches. Worse, it made sex a planned activity; any spontaneity was gone. Caitlin believed that this would have been difficult but acceptable if it were not for her own sexual problems following cancer treatment. Their attempts at intercourse, whether prolonged with or without Viagra, were painful for her and frustrating for them both. "A few nights ago, I finally had to ask him to stop. I felt terrible, he felt terrible, and the whole episode was a disaster."

The first step for Caitlin and her husband was admitting there was a problem. The second step was finding a way to talk about it without shame or blame. They felt that meeting with me, in a neutral and professional setting, would make discussing this feel safer. We talked together about the physical realities for each and the fact that these were separate from their love for each other and their wish to maintain an active sexual connection. We talked about sexual pleasure without intercourse, about strategies to enjoy intercourse with less pressure and pain for her, and the overriding value of their wish to be close. Not surprisingly, when Caitlin checked in with me some weeks later, she reported that matters were greatly improved. Simply talking together had relieved the personal pressure each had been feeling. They were now experimenting with other kinds of physical closeness and sexual activity and were incorporating the use of Viagra as one possibility when they were making love.

Breast cancer treatment often wreaks havoc on sexuality. It is certainly never a sexual aid. Women who have had a mastectomy, with or without reconstruction, may have the hardest time feeling desirable and womanly. *May* is the operative word here. Many women feel like Hannah, who said, "My husband always tells me that I am beautiful. I have never felt disfigured or less sexy because I have one breast." But others cannot bear to look at their flat chests and their scars even months after the surgery. Some, like Barbara, say, "Every morning when I awaken and remember my mastectomies, I feel that I have lost my compass. It takes a few minutes to find due north." Even those who have had less-disfiguring surgery may still feel that their breasts are ugly. Swollen after radiation, smaller because tissue has been excised, scarred, lumpy from scar tissue—breasts look different, and even worse, they may feel different.

Women who have had mastectomies, with or without reconstruction, are numb in the chest area. The sensation of having no sensation is especially upsetting during sex. Some also find that their chest walls remain hypersensitive, so being touched may be painful. Those who have had lumpectomies may also have areas of numbness and areas where sensation has changed. These changes may include hypersensitivity, chronic soreness or even pain when touched, and just plain "oddness." The skin may look and feel different to your touch. The best advice is to remember yet again that time will help. You will become accustomed to these areas of numbness, and they will feel increasingly like you. Janet commented: "I used to feel that an alien had landed on my chest and taken away any feelings. Now I know it's just good old me."

For all women, the reminder of what has been lost is poignant. Even if you don't feel that you have experienced actual physical changes in your body, you may well find that your sense of yourself has changed. Breasts are important to us as women in so many ways. It is a cliché to talk about the value our society places on breasts, and it is impossible to open a magazine or go to a movie without being reminded of this. Women, especially those who have lost a breast, talk about how painful it can be to watch lovemaking scenes in movies or even to read about them in novels. In contrast, several women have reminded me about Amazon women, warriors who chose to have a breast amputated to better position a bow. This image of strength can be powerful.

Losing a breast or having a very changed breast is a genuine loss. It is normal to grieve this body change, and it is also normal to gradually come to a place of acceptance. Kay, who had bilateral mastectomies, said several years later that she still awakens each morning and is hit with a wave of sadness as she remembers what has happened. The difference now is that the wave is less intense and shorter.

Margery, a fifty-year-old divorced consultant, said, "Until I had my son when I was thirty-five, I had a sexy body, primarily because of my breasts. Husbands and lovers would always say 'Great tits!' I considered them my best erogenous zone. Even after nursing my son and a biopsy scar from a benign lump, I still had great breasts. And for all of my twenties, thirties, and forties, I loved sex. Since my surgery, I hate the way my breast looks and I have zero interest in sex."

She went on to talk about the impact of this change on her social life. "Maybe if I were in a marriage or a relationship that began before breast cancer, things would be different. As it is, I am afraid to take chances, afraid of rejection and failure in a new relationship. So I forge ahead in other areas of my life, sometimes still stunned and sad that the magic of intimacy no longer seems available. At other times I can be accepting and just grateful to be alive and to have the love of my family and friends."

A vital first step in regaining your sexual health is accepting, appreciating, even learning to honor your body. The psychological component of this process is enormous. You may feel that your body, especially your breast, has betrayed you. You may find it very difficult to trust your physical responses and instincts, which can make it hard to relax enough to feel and enjoy pleasurable sensations. Time will alleviate this to a degree, but you can try to speed up the timetable. As trivial as it may seem, it will help to pay attention to all of your senses and your body as you work toward becoming comfortable again inside your skin.

Think about all the things, not just sexual, that give you physical or sensual pleasure: bubble baths, silk lingerie, scented body lotions, back rubs. Expand your thoughts to consider different kinds of pleasure: flowers on the table, the feeling of grass on your bare feet, chocolate. Think, too, of well-used and tired muscles after a day of skiing or a long hike, water from a hot shower beating on your shoulders, and the smell of bread baking. You may find it helpful to make a list, perhaps separating the pleasures by senses (visual, tactile, or smell) or by their value to you. Once you have this list, use it! Make sure that every day you care for yourself in at least one way that will give you pleasure and stimulate one of your senses.

Gradually it will be important to become more focused on sexual sensation and response. There are a number of sexual sensate exercises that you or you and your partner can try. For example, you can take turns spending ten minutes giving each other a massage. You are directed to use only your hands in as many ways as possible. Try different lotions or oils. Try playing soft music or lighting candles as background. Keep your hands only on the back; nowhere else is allowed! Another simple exercise is using as many different things as you can find to stroke each other's back and legs. Again, set the stage with music and soft lighting. Then, in ten-minute turns, stroke each other with a feather, a silk scarf, something cool, something warm, something rough, whatever you can imagine. Remember, you are restricted to only backs and legs! The goal of any of these exercises is to help you learn to focus on sensation without any pressure of sexual performance or intercourse. More information about them can be found in the reference materials noted in the "Resources" section of this book.

Even if you become comfortable in your own skin and are at least thinking in a positive and sensual way about sexual activity, you may find that you are experiencing physical difficulties that interfere with your pleasure. Chemotherapy, especially if it produces a chemical menopause, changes your hormonal makeup. We know that it generally slows down your metabolism and your body, and your sexual responsiveness and your libido are part of that slowdown.

You probably find it harder and slower to become

aroused and even harder and slower to achieve orgasm. I realize it can be frustrating to even think about orgasm this way, as a project, but I promise you it will help. The chairs in my office have wooden arms, and more than one woman has stroked them and described her previously responsive erogenous zones as feeling the same way now that the wood does. Some women find that regular masturbation helps reclaim libido, arousal, and even improved lubrication. All women experience physiological changes following menopause and the loss of their previous estrogen levels. It is likely that a chemically induced menopause, so abrupt and sometimes so premature, makes these changes even more intense.

The loss of estrogen with menopause is a major problem for some women. Estrogen loss can result in hot flashes, vaginal dryness, pain during intercourse caused by the thinning of the vaginal walls, and a decrease in bone density that may lead to osteoporosis.

There is ongoing controversy about the use of hormone-replacement therapy (HRT) for all women, not just for those who have had breast cancer. While this issue is not likely to be fully resolved for some time, if at all, the advisability and safety of HRT for all postmenopausal women is uncertain. There has been a recent major change in prevailing medical opinion. During the summer of 2002, the NIH actually halted an ongoing landmark clinical trial examining the value of HRT for all women, because of the evidence of possible negative effects. For women who have had breast cancer, HRT is thought to be even less wise. Since breast cancer is a disease that is often mediated by estrogens (that is, if the breast cancer cells are estrogen-receptor positive), most oncologists believe that it is unwise, and maybe even unsafe, for a woman who has been treated for breast cancer to take HRT. The concern is that if any remaining microscopic breast cancer cells are lying dormant in the body, exposure to estrogens might stimulate them to grow. It is worth repeating this information because, while this is a theoretical worry, it is an extremely important one, and the stakes are very high.

Are there ever circumstances when taking estrogen after breast cancer is a wise decision? This question can be answered only after thoughtful and thorough discussions with your oncologist and your gynecologist. It will be necessary to consider the bothersome symptoms you are experiencing and whether there are nonestrogen alternatives that might be helpful. For example, severe hot flashes may be ameliorated by a low dose of a commonly used antidepressant, Effexor. Vaginal dryness and dyspareunia (pain during intercourse) can often be helped by lubricants, discussed later in this chapter. Diminishing bone density can be treated with exercise, calcium supplements, and sometimes with the addition of bisphosphonate drugs such as Fosamax and Actonel.

However, there are instances in which some symptoms or problems do not respond to these measures. If this is your situation, you may be faced with an agonizing decision—do you take estrogen, with its unknown but possible risks, to alleviate your symptoms? You will have to consider how impaired your sexuality is, how much your relationship is affected, and how much risk and attendant anxiety you can tolerate. If you and your doctors do decide to use estrogen, the best alternative is to choose the method that

offers the least systemic exposure: namely, estrogen deliv-
ered intravaginally either through the insertion of a tiny
ring that slowly releases the hormone over time (E string)
or by the topical application of a hormone cream. Although
a tiny amount of estrogen is absorbed into the bloodstream
through the lining of the vaginal walls, most of the drug's effect is local. Thus, vaginal dryness and painful intercourse
are likely to be markedly improved. It must be emphasized,
however, that the absolute safety of using the E string or
topical low-dose estrogen in this way has not been deter-
mined, so this is a decision to be made with great care and
in discussion with your doctors.

As noted earlier, estrogen is not the only hormone that
affects sexual response in women. Testosterone, though
usually associated with men, is the major female sex hormone affecting libido. Low testosterone levels—also an as-
pect of menopause—can cause declines in arousal, genital
sensation, libido, and orgasm. Testosterone deficiency is
also associated with a diminished sense of well-being (something that can be difficult to tease out from all the other factors in your post-cancer experience) and sometimes with
the thinning of pubic hair. It is possible to have a blood test
that evaluates hormone levels, and your doctor may find
that your testosterone level is below normal. If so, a small
dose of testosterone might indeed stimulate your sex drive,
but there are potential undesirable side effects from testosterone, such as developing male secondary sexual characteristics like facial hair and a deepening voice. And as with
estrogen, it is unclear whether testosterone is safe for
women who have had breast cancer. This is a complex decision that must be made jointly with your doctor.

Depression can also be a major factor in the loss of libido. As mentioned in Chapter 3, many women are at least sad and worried, and sometimes depressed, after cancer. It is impossible to feel very sexy when these are your overriding emotions. Fatigue is another symptom of depression, as well as a frequent companion of cancer treatment and recovery. When these feelings consume you, sex is not going to be high on your priority list.

If you find yourself still mired in depression after a few months have passed, it is time to ask for help. Loss of interest in sex is one of the classic symptoms of depression, and you may in fact identify this problem by recognizing this loss of interest. Chapter 17 discusses helpful resources for dealing with depression. There are differences between a clinical depression that may be helped by medication and a sadness that is caused by real-life circumstances. The latter is what is called a reactive depression and is the experience of many women after cancer; it will slowly improve as her emotional and physical recovery progresses. Drugs won't help and they won't speed up the natural timetable. Any decision to take an antidepressant should be made in consultation with a therapist who is experienced in working with breast cancer patients. It is extremely important to sort out the depression/sadness that is a normal part of the cancer experience from a clinical depression, which is a separate disorder that *will* respond to medications. You should also be aware that many of the more popular antidepressants, such as Prozac and Zoloft, can cause diminished libido as a side effect.

Even worse than difficulties with libido and orgasm can be pain during intercourse. Diminished levels of estrogen cause thinning and shortening of the vaginal walls, which makes penetration very uncomfortable. Tamoxifen results in more lubrication and comfort for some women, but for others the same drug seems to enhance dryness. If you are experiencing discomfort or pain during intercourse and if maintaining an active sex life that includes penetration is important to you, you must attend to this problem as soon as possible. Each time that you have painful intercourse will make the psychological problem worse. This kind of conditioning and negative reinforcement has to be addressed quickly.

Vaginal dryness is the most common reason for discomfort or pain during intercourse. It can be awkward or embarrassing to talk about this with your partner and to include lubrication in your sexual foreplay. However, wetter is definitely better, and you will both benefit greatly from the use of lubricants. Try including it in your touching and exploration of each other rather than leaving an application to the moment before penetration. Spread it around your genital area as well as your partner's. You can both put some on your fingers or hands and gently touch each other; the sensations will be stimulating, and the moisture will help you move on to satisfying intercourse. There are many over-the-counter products available at pharmacies; some of the better-known ones are Astroglide, Moist Again, Replens, Surgilube, and K-Y Jelly. Try several. Replens works slightly differently from others; try applying it three times weekly rather than at times when you are about to engage in sexual activity. (Applying Replens two days before a scheduled gynecological examination may also help to make that more comfortable.) There is also some research suggesting that the topical use of Retin-A vaginally may help. Ask your gynecologist. In addition, there are two surprising products that help many women with lubrication and are available inexpensively and with no embarrassment at the supermarket: try plain yogurt or canola oil.

In addition to dryness, loss of elasticity in the vaginal walls can also cause painful intercourse. This is less easily managed, but regular use of Replens may be useful because it helps the cells of the vagina retain moisture and thus seem thicker. It also helps to work on gently stretching your vagina. You can use your fingers, especially while sitting in a warm bath, or you can buy dildos or vaginal dilators (available with a prescription at most pharmacies). Make sure that anything you are inserting into your vagina is clean, and use a lubricant or do this in the bathtub.

Position during intercourse can make a major difference in comfort. The standard missionary position may be the least comfortable, but if this is your preferred position, try putting a pillow under your hips to change the angle. Experiment with several options: spooning (your partner lying behind you and entering from the rear), being on top, or sitting on your partner so that you control the depth of thrust. Try changing leg positions and tensing and relaxing your vagina during intercourse. Another trick may be to bring your partner to orgasm, either by hand or orally, before you attempt intercourse. If he can achieve a second erection, it will probably be slightly smaller and his urgency will be diminished. One irony of nature is that men, as they become aroused, want faster and harder sensations while women often want softer and gentler ones. Be aware, too, that position and angle will affect your partner's experience. In order to maintain an erection and achieve an orgasm, men usually need to experience the pleasing sensation of contact between the penis and the walls of the vagina. Different positions bring different degrees of contact, and it may be important for you to communicate clearly with each other about your experiences. Finding ways to please you both may take experimentation and time, but you will find them.

Resuming an active and loving sexual connection is worth the effort. Julie, a physician in her early forties, described the initial experience of having sex with her husband after her mastectomy as being "as awkward as the first time. Even though I have been having sex with this man for twenty years, it felt completely strange and new." Clearly her changed body itself felt strange and new to her, and her own uncertainty affected him, too.

There are other stories and experiences that are completely positive. One of my patients is married to a very tall, muscular, long-haired, tattooed biker. The first time they made love after her mastectomy, he gently laid his head on her scar and said, "Now I can lie closer to your heart."

As you know, the introduction of Viagra has made a major impact on men's sexual functioning. There are studies now looking at the value of Viagra for women. Another possibility is Viacream, a nonprescription product sold through the Internet, which is applied topically to the genital area. The active ingredients in Viacream are menthol USP and L-arginine, an amino acid found in dairy products. It stimulates the sensitive tissues and is said to provide women with a heightened sexual sensitivity and responsiveness, so it may enhance or ease the achievement of orgasm.

If you are experiencing difficulties with sexual arousal or orgasm, it is worth speaking with your doctor. Do not be surprised if your oncologist is not well informed about these concerns. You may do better to speak with your gynecologist, to a medical specialist in women's sexual functioning, or to a sex therapist. These therapists are mental-health practitioners—psychiatrists, psychologists, or social workers—who have special training in the treatment of sexual dysfunction. You can locate a certified sex therapist by calling the American Association of Sex Educators, Counselors, and Therapists at 319-895-8407; they also have a helpful Web site. Before making an appointment, however, have a telephone conversation to ascertain that the therapist also has experience treating women who have had cancer. You can expect a sex therapist to assess both your relationship and your sexual skills. She will talk with you about normal sexual function and the impact of your cancer and treatment on it, give you advice and practical suggestions that are both medically and psychologically appropriate, and work to enhance communication and pleasure for you and your partner. There are also books that can help you do some of this work on your own; for suggestions, see the "Resources" section.

Special Concerns of Single Women

Women who are not in a committed relationship at the time of their breast cancer diagnosis and treatment may experience heightened concerns about sexuality. It is never easy to manage the singles dating scene, and having been treated for breast cancer is certainly not an advantage. In addition to whatever concerns and difficulties about dating you had prior to cancer, you are probably wondering whether anyone could possibly find you attractive and desirable now. The short answer to this question is an emphatic "Yes!"

Several of my single patients have described their cancer experience as functioning like advanced radar. As simple as this sounds, it is a quick and useful way to separate the men from the boys (or the women from the girls). Any partner worth having will have the necessary maturity to accept you as you now are. The sole exception to this rule, in all honesty, may be men who have lost their lover or wife to breast cancer. It is understandable that they may feel they cannot expose themselves to the possibility of another such loss. Others, however, may bring a special empathy to your situation because of their prior experiences and be eager to know you better.

If you are apprehensive about how to begin to meet men or how to talk with them about your cancer, you may find it very helpful to talk with other unmarried breast cancer survivors who have faced the same situation. There are two general areas of concern: your own emotional vulnerability and the worry that a man may perceive you as "damaged goods," and anxiety about how to begin an intimate relationship given your changed body and sexual responses.

Because you are especially concerned about new relationships, you will take your time. Even if in the past you sometimes participated in one-night stands or brief, intense relationships, these are not behaviors you will be considering now. It is definitely not necessary to tell someone about your cancer at your first meeting. Remember that you are a complete and valuable woman. Cancer is one part of your history and so part of who you are—but *only* one part. Obviously, as you come to know each other, the time will come when you will need to talk with him about it. Choose the moment carefully, and do not wait to have this conversation until you are within moments of becoming sexually intimate.

The biggest challenge for single women is finding the self-confidence and the courage to begin to be open to a new relationship. In coping with the many challenges of recovery, reclaiming your social/sexual self will be one of the larger ones. Beginning to date always means taking risks, and because you are already feeling vulnerable, those risks will feel greater. Exposing yourself for the first time to a potential partner is never easy. When the time comes, revealing your changed body will be even harder. It will help if you talk with him openly about your concerns, how shy you are feeling, how difficult it may have been to accept your body after treatment. Describe what your body looks and feels like; try to be very clear so that he will not be surprised by a scar, an odd shape, a missing breast.

It is likely that you will find that he, like your other friends, is unsophisticated about breast cancer and will need information from you. You must tell him honestly about what happened, how your body has changed, and what your feelings and worries are as you move toward the future. Since most women who have had breast cancer go on to live long and healthy lives, you can absolutely be reassuring about that. Articulating your feelings aloud always makes them easier to bear. Remind yourself of what you have accomplished and mastered. You are no stranger to courage. I have never heard of a man who fled a new relationship when the cancer was disclosed. To the contrary, I have heard lovely stories about sensitive men who said, "We all have scars. Some are more visible than others." Or, just as movingly, "I just wish I had known you then so you could have leaned on me."

IO

Fertility and Pregnancy

After breast cancer, some women are left with a particularly painful and ambiguous life question. The American Cancer Society estimates that at least twenty-six thousand women of childbearing age are diagnosed with breast cancer each year in the United States. Worry and grief about the possible loss of fertility and the chance to bear children are sometimes the most anguishing aspects of this experience.

There is never a good or right time to have cancer, but developing it as a young woman is especially hard. While your peers are thinking about babies, you are forced to think about chemotherapy. While your peers are planning their families, you are terrified that you may not survive to have a child.

If you have not had children or have not had all the children you planned, you will be very worried about your fertility and about the wisdom of a future pregnancy. Women who have already had a child but hoped for a larger family can be just as sad as women who are childless. Even those who do not expect to have children are often devastated by the possibility of treatment-caused infertility. Part of this pain has to do with being deprived of choice, with the absence of control, the fact of yet one more very major loss caused by cancer. Coming to grips with the possible end of your dreams of childbearing may mean having to deal all over again with grief and rage over your cancer diagnosis. This is yet one more thing, and a very important one, that cancer has stolen from you.

Cancer has completely rearranged your life plan. If this is your situation, it is likely that you will be thinking about the question of a future pregnancy and whether it is safe or even possible for you, as well as the question of adoption or other ways of building a family.

If, after careful consideration with your husband or partner, you know that you want to bear a child, you must now consider the physical and medical implications of a pregnancy. The traditional wisdom had been that it was unwise for a woman to become pregnant after breast cancer. In the early years of my practice, I vividly remember hearing doctors present this strong opinion to their patients. Before the widespread use of adjuvant treatment for early breast cancer, survival rates were significantly lower than they are now, and doctors were even more apprehensive about their patients' future health.

Today, however, oncologists believe that pregnancy following breast cancer—especially after the passage of several healthy years—will not increase the likelihood of recurrence. Most doctors do suggest that their patients wait at least three years, and sometimes five, following their breast cancer before becoming pregnant. This advice is based on the fact that most aggressive breast cancers recur within that time period. There have been a number of studies looking at the recurrence rates among women who do or do not become pregnant following breast cancer. Large retrospective studies have indicated there is no higher risk of recurrence among women who go on to have a pregnancy three or more years beyond their initial diagnosis. However, there are concerns about the design of these studies, and the bottom line is that no one knows with complete certainty about the impact of pregnancy on breast-cancer survivors.

Admittedly, being told that you should wait three to five years before becoming pregnant can seem endless, now that you are finally done with treatment and eager to get on with your life! But since waiting is inevitable, it is advisable to use a barrier form of birth control during the time that you are trying to avoid a pregnancy. You should not assume that because you are not menstruating (and it can take a year or more for your periods to resume after chemotherapy) that you are not fertile.

One thing you can do during these years that may help is to talk with your doctor about meeting with an infertility specialist and having an evaluation. Even though you do not want to become pregnant now, it may be helpful later to have the baseline information in place. You can also use this time to explore adoption and other alternatives. The more information you have, the better prepared you will be to proceed when the right time comes.

If you are considering adopting a child, you must also

contend with the reluctance of some adoption agencies to consider the applications of women who have had cancer. This would be a good time to investigate different agencies and their positions on adoption by parents who have had serious illness. You will need strong supporting letters from your doctors and you may need to wait a specified period of time before you can apply. I have known a number of women who, both through agencies and through private adoptions, have adopted children after having had breast cancer. Complicated though the process may be, this is not an impossible option.

Soon after the end of her chemotherapy, Susan, a thirty-two-year-old attorney, and her husband decided to research other ways to have a child. By speaking with infertility specialists, they found a wealth of information about surrogate mothers, egg donations, and other techniques that might help them now or later. "We may decide to go ahead and have another woman carry a baby using my husband's sperm, or we may wait for me," Susan said, "but it is enormously helpful to be doing something and to realize we have some options."

The first issue, of course, is your fertility. The reason that chemotherapy sometimes ends a woman's menses and fertility is simple. You may recall that a baby girl is born with all of the eggs in her infant ovaries that she will ever have. After she begins to menstruate, approximately fifty of those eggs begin to mature each month, although usually only one matures fully and becomes viable. As the years pass, the lifetime supply of eggs diminishes. Chemotherapy, in killing all fast-growing cells, destroys the follicles that protect and nurture those eggs and damages normal hormonal cycles. Since younger women have more remaining eggs, they have a greater chance than older women that some of them will recover and be viable in the future.

You may have been lucky and had the chance to discuss these issues with your medical oncologist before your treatment. Some oncologists, aware that you hope to be able to have a baby in the future, may suggest a course of adjuvant chemotherapy that uses drugs that may spare ovarian function. Others may administer a medication, Lupron, in the hope of protecting future ovarian function. Lupron shuts down the ovaries temporarily, creating in effect a reversible menopause. When the medication is stopped, menses are likely to resume. Alternatively, a woman may choose to store her eggs in a manner similar to (but much more complicated than) sperm banking for male cancer patients.

In women who are nearing the end of their fertile years, chemotherapy usually terminates ovulation and menstruation. Women in their twenties and early thirties are likely to regain their periods post-chemotherapy. Women in between—that is, those in their mid-thirties to mid-forties—are in an ambiguous zone. In order to best treat your cancer and reduce your risk of recurrence, your doctor may feel it is wise to shut down your cycles and decrease the estrogen in your body. This is especially true for women who have had estrogen-receptor-positive breast cancers. Since some younger women continue to menstruate while taking tamoxifen, you may also be advised to receive Lupron shots to temporarily shut down your ovaries.

Aromatase inhibitors, the other possible hormone treatments for women with estrogen-receptor-positive breast cancers, are given only to postmenopausal women.

For younger women, the recommendation to take tamoxifen after completing chemotherapy presents a special dilemma. Tamoxifen can stop the menses permanently, depending on the individual and on her age. Knowing that the older you are, the less certain you can be that your periods—and your fertility—will resume when the tamoxifen therapy ends, what do you do? You face a dilemma if you are advised to take this drug for five years to minimize the risk of recurrence or the development of cancer in your other breast. You want to do all you can to prevent any more cancer, but you know that fertility declines with age, and five years is a long time when your biological clock is ticking.

Obviously an initial step can be to find out whether you are still fertile following chemotherapy. The answer would seem to be that if your periods return, you can still conceive. This is frequently but not always true; we all know of healthy menstruating women who have not had cancer but who have difficulty achieving a pregnancy. There are a couple of standard blood tests that can give you information about your fertility. The first measures the amount of estradiol, the most important female hormone, in your blood. If your ovaries are no longer functioning, estradiol will not be present. The second possible test confirms the levels of serum LH (luteinizing hormone) and FSH (follicle-stimulating hormone) in your blood. Your doctor can tell by the levels of these hormones whether your ovaries are functioning or whether you are in menopause.

All these factors that may affect your fertility are related to the treatment of your known breast cancer. There are two main concerns about pregnancy after breast cancer.

The first is the possibility that the hormones of pregnancy might stimulate the growth of any cancer cells that are left in your body. Pregnancy does not cause cancer, but its hormones may hasten a recurrence. The second is worry about your continuing good health. A recurrence of breast cancer during pregnancy would be an anguishing situation. Depending on the stage of pregnancy, you would have to face questions about termination and about the impact of any cancer treatments on the fetus. Even worse is the worry about the possibility of your premature death, leaving a young child to be raised by others.

As hard as it is to face it, the single most important consideration is your survival. The people who love you care most about *you,* not about an unborn child. It would be foolhardy to knowingly do anything that would reduce the chances that you will live a long and healthy life.

There are both medical and existential issues involved in this dilemma. Any woman who has had breast cancer must consider the serious question: Is bringing a child into the world or into my family a responsible act when I cannot be sure I will live to raise him or her? Obviously no woman is guaranteed sound health in which to raise her children, but you are in a different category from those who have not received a diagnosis of a potentially life-threatening illness.

It is imperative that you and your husband or partner consider this decision and all the possible scenarios very seriously. Everyone lives with the risk of sudden death from accidents, natural disasters, and medical emergencies. If your husband is an older man or has had medical problems himself, you may have already worried about the possibility that he would die prematurely and leave you to raise your children alone. Now you must add to this the chance that he might be the one left behind and even that your children might be orphaned.

Choosing to have a baby after breast cancer forces you to be a very responsible expectant parent. The same questions that all parents must grapple with assume additional importance when you are painfully aware of your mortality. Do you have family or very close friends whom you could count on to help your husband raise children as you would wish them to be raised? Will there be adequate financial resources to meet your children's needs and education? It is not enough for the two of you to have this intimate conversation. You also need to talk with the family members or friends whom you think of as guardians of your future children. Are they willing and able to make this commitment to you?

Having gone through breast cancer, you are probably more committed than ever to living your life fully and joyfully, and you may feel that being a mother is a vital part of that life. The ticking biological clock that you barely heard before your cancer may now be chiming loudly. Even if you were not considering parenthood before cancer, you may be longing for it now. The passion for life that helped you through the months of treatment may drive you now toward creating and shepherding a new life.

Women who have been treated with chemotherapy for breast cancer often worry about the possible impact of that treatment on a future pregnancy. It is reassuring to know that all the available data suggest that previous chemotherapy for breast cancer has no impact on the development of a healthy baby. If you have had radiation treatment to your breast, it is likely that breast will not produce milk to nurse a baby, but your untreated breast can produce enough to nourish your child.

Still, the decision to have a child is a very personal and individual one. You and your husband or partner must talk with your doctor about your particular kind of cancer, your treatments, and the recurrence rates and risks that statistically you are facing. You need to ask about all the research in these areas and how your doctor thinks you fit into the findings. With all of the information you can garner, you are then able to make the best possible decision for yourself and for your family. If your head and your heart encourage you to pursue this dream, do it!

II

—

Children

If you are a mother it is very likely that, in the first blinding moments of knowing you had breast cancer, your heart and your thoughts went to your children. It was certainly my instant reaction: the heart-stopping fear of leaving my daughters motherless. Because of my divorce from their father, I was raising them alone. He was rarely present, and my fiancé was far too new in their lives to be a paternal figure. All of us privately acknowledge our shortcomings as parents; we appreciate that we mother or father our children imperfectly. In the words of the Episcopal Church's Book of Common Prayer, we know that *We have left undone those things which we ought to have done; and we have done those things which we ought not have done.* But whatever our inadequacies, we always expect to give our children safe passage to adulthood. We assume we will be there to shield them, protect them, nurture and love them until they can stand sturdily alone. For me, hearing my diagnosis meant having to recognize that I might be the instrument—unwittingly and unwillingly, but the instrument nonetheless—of the worst thing that I could imagine befalling my daughters: losing their mother.

At that time, they were at very different moments in their lives, so their reactions and adjustments were different and age-appropriate. Katharine was a junior in college, halfway across the country. Because both her grandmothers had also had breast cancer, her immediate and natural reaction was to worry about her own future health. "What does this mean for me?" she asked, and since I, too, worried about this, all I could do was murmur reassurances and privately weep. At twenty, she was working to separate from me, to establish her independence and to create a fulfilling adult life. She was mature enough to understand the possible implications for her own future and secure enough in herself and in our relationship to speak out about her fear. In that first conversation, she needed to be told she would be fine and that I was likely to be fine, and to be reminded that one of her grandmothers, my mother, appeared to have been cured of the disease. But despite these reassurances, neither of us could forget that her other grandmother had died of it.

My younger daughter, Julia, was in seventh grade, and her first response was the bluntest question of all: "Will you die?" This was quickly followed by "Will you lose your breast?" and "Will you lose your hair?" I told her, as I had told so many mothers to tell their children, that I would not die. No one ever drops dead of breast cancer, and if the future brought recurrence and the prospect of eventual death, there would be plenty of time to talk about it then. At this moment of diagnosis, she needed to be told I would be well. Because of my work life and our dinner-table conversations that often included cancer, she was aware that breast cancer treatment sometimes meant losing a breast and losing one's hair. I did not need to have a mastectomy, but I knew that I would lose my hair, so I answered those questions honestly. Then we held each other close and wept.

As time passed, all three of us found ways to manage the fear and the sadness and to support one another. Two months into my chemotherapy, even though I was exhausted and feeling ill, I forced myself to keep a commitment to give a talk in Nebraska. The flights were delayed; I arrived late at the conference; I barely remember the talk or how it was received. My primary reason for making the trip was to stop on the way home to visit with Katharine in Minnesota. Although I spent much of the weekend napping, it was important for her to see me and for us to be together. It was also that visit on her own turf that showed me how deeply she was affected by my illness. Although she had quickly resumed her busy college schedule and seemed to be doing well, her room was filled with notes and cards from her friends. She, too, had needed support and help, and they were responding.

Julia, of course, was living at home, so her daily life was directly affected by my treatment. After the crisis of a canceled trip to Disney World at the time of my surgery, we tried hard to enable her to resume and maintain her usual routines. She continued to ask for rides, for help with homework, for trips to the mall, and I was usually able to respond.

But still I remember lying on my bed early one Friday evening and telling her that I could not, just could not, drive her and her friends to the movies. There was a predictable spurt of anger; then she quickly made other arrangements. I, of course, felt guilty and sad and overwhelmed by worry about how she could manage without me.

As I had advised countless other mothers to do, I tried to involve her and engage her help in appropriate ways. Like any teenager, this did not mean that she offered to do the laundry or load the dishwasher, but she did discover one way to be enormously helpful. I had great difficulty with the Cytoxan tablets that were part of my chemotherapy regimen. By the second cycle, I was dealing with anticipatory nausea that arose just from looking at the pill bottle. Julia came into the room one day as I was struggling to take the day's pills. She took them from me and suggested that I imagine they were mint M&M's; she described at length the texture and taste and sensation of the candies melting in my mouth as I swallowed the pills. This imagery and distraction were so valuable that she began to hand me the pills each day (it helped if I never had to touch or look at them) and to create a different image for me to focus on. We went through many candies and many berries and came back to the mint M&M's on the worst days.

It is very likely that your children will have adjusted quickly and managed reasonably well during your months of treatment. I and colleagues in my hospital's Department of Psychiatry worked on a longitudinal study of the reactions of children to a mother's breast cancer, and we have found, over and over, that children who are given age-appropriate information and whose routines remain consistent do very well. Indeed, their mothers say that it sometimes seems as if the children actually forget about the cancer and so are startled when they catch a glimpse of a bald head or are told of a doctor's appointment. They do not really forget, of course, nor are they in denial. It is simply that their healthy defenses are working well, protecting them as they go about their daily business of growing up.

In fact, mothers undergoing treatment often report that they are hurt by their children's apparent indifference to their cancer. We know that it is natural for children to be extremely self-centered. As long as they feel safe and cared for, they are usually able to function normally within their family and in their world. Your cancer is not and should not be the priority for them that it is for you. Nor is it surprising that these same dynamics persist after treatment is finished. As long as you seem to be doing well, they will, too.

Here is an example of how much a child, even in a family where cancer is discussed openly, can manage to not deal with it. Sue Ellen told the story of being out to dinner with her family several years after the completion of her chemotherapy. Her youngest child was only two during her treatment, but the family had always been open and honest about it, and he had not been sheltered from her experience. But when, during dinner, she made a casual reference to "when I was being treated for breast cancer . . ." he stood up abruptly, knocking over his chair, and yelled, "*You* had breast cancer?" She was stunned that he seemed to have entirely repressed the year. As we talked about the incident, she gradually appreciated that his "forgetting" her cancer was actually a sign of his sturdy mental health and her family's wise management of her illness as an unhappy moment in life but not as her whole life.

Like that boy, preschool children are likely to have no real memory of your time in treatment. If you have no older children, this situation presents an odd choice. Assuming that you stay well, you could opt not to mention your cancer to your children until they are much older, though at some point they certainly will need to know your medical history in order to take adequate care of themselves. My strong suggestion, however, is to mention your cancer now and then in a matter-of-fact way. Tell a story about something that happened during your months of treatment. Reminisce about the nurse you liked so much. Talk about a friend whom you met in the oncology waiting room. Your children will take their emotional cues from you and, as long as you are talking about cancer calmly, they will not be upset. But never mentioning it shrouds it in secrecy and makes it seem a very bad and frightening thing. It is also very likely that your children will hear it mentioned in the context of someone else's diagnosis or your own follow-up appointments. If your cancer history is part of the backdrop of their lives, along with an uncle's car accident or the death of a family pet or even a trip you once took before they were born, this will put it in perspective for them.

Older children will, of course, remember. Even though it may seem to you that they have forgotten, you can be certain that your cancer is an important part of their emotional lives. School-age children are apt to behave as though it never happened, and this is a sign of their doing well, but it does not mean that their antennae are not poised or that they are oblivious to your conversations or feelings. They are listening and watching, but what they observe will not be emotionally charged as long as you seem well. Generally it is a good idea to casually mention at dinner that you had a doctor's appointment today and everything was fine, or that you have decided to donate your wig to the hospital so another woman can use it, or that you had lunch today with a friend you met during radiation therapy. Don't be surprised if your children don't respond at all and the conversation moves quickly to another subject. The point is to be matter-of-fact, to include your cancer recovery in your life along with everything else that is going on. The objective is to make the cancer part of the frame of their lives but not the central picture.

Intriguingly, many women can feel especially hurt by their adolescent daughters' apparent indifference to their breast cancer, as if a daughter on the cusp of womanhood should surely be more empathetic and involved. But we all know that adolescents—sons *and* daughters—are notoriously self-absorbed as they work to separate from their parents. This normal developmental phase takes different paths in different children. Thus, some teenagers become active in breast cancer causes, choosing to walk in fund-raising events and even planning breast cancer-awareness sessions at school or in the community. Many, however, have no interest in activities like these; indeed, they may be loath to publicly identify themselves as the son or daughter of a breast cancer survivor. This is perfectly fine and entirely normal. The important thing is to allow your children, of any age, to deal with your cancer and their fears about it, each in his or her own way. Some children cope by taking in the experience little by little, allowing only as much as they can tolerate at any given time.

The advice about including your cancer in your normal conversations is equally important with your adolescent children. Continue, as always, to answer their questions honestly. It might be wise, especially the first year when the experience is so recent, to mention that your checkups and your annual mammogram went well. But do not count on much of a reaction. Your teenagers may share your elation or may just shrug. Either way, though, they have certainly heard you and have had welcome news.

It is likely that sometime in the future your seemingly uninterested child will talk with you about how scared she or he was. It may take the safety of time before children can even truly admit this fright to themselves. It may also be that news of the diagnosis of a friend's mother or someone else they know will stir up all of those latent fears about your own illness, perhaps provoking an intense reaction. This, too, is normal. If it happens, encourage them to talk about how they felt, and let them know that you were scared, too. Make sure to remind them that you are doing fine now, that your doctors are following you carefully, and that you will always be honest with them. Children may worry that you will keep bad news from them, and it is important to be clear that you will not do this. That way, when you have not told them of a problem, they can be confident that there is none.

If your children ask you to reassure them of your good health—"Are you cured now, Mommy?"—be honest but lean toward the positive. Adolescent and adult children could be told: "I'm doing fine now and am really hopeful that I will stay well." This gives them an opportunity, if they want it, to ask for additional information, but it also gives them permission to take your answer and be satisfied. With younger children, your answer should be a more emphatic "Yes." Again, worries about recurrence belong to you and the adults who love you. If you should have to deal with cancer again, there will be plenty of time then to talk about it.

Judith told the following story about her son, who was eight at the time of her diagnosis and is now fourteen, a high-school freshman. "Last week, for the first time ever, he started talking with me about what had happened. Maybe it was because his friend's father was just diagnosed with colon cancer. Anyway, he said, 'My friends were shocked when I mentioned that my mom had had cancer. I thought it was something everyone's mom went through. I thought that your hair falling out and you coming home from work early and throwing up was normal.' Well, we did try to keep things normal for him. I can't tell you how many soccer games I suffered through, nauseated with the sun beating down on my balding scalp, and acting like nothing was going on. . . ."

However, it is also advisable to be alert to the possibility that a child is reacting to your cancer through anxieties, whether specific fears or a more generalized worry, that do not on the surface seem to be clearly related to it. Thus, for example, a small child might become afraid of thunderstorms, or an older child might suddenly be worried about a myriad of issues. While these behaviors may indeed be reflective of other concerns, always consider the possibility that your child *is* actually worried about you and your health and is displacing that anxiety onto another problem. If you think this is possible, ask him or her about it directly. You can say something like, "As I listen to you worry about your teacher getting sick and leaving school, I can't help but wonder if you are also worrying about me. We all remember that I had breast cancer last year, and all of us think and worry about it sometimes."

Err on the side of staying concerned about your children. I want to again emphasize that most youngsters whose mothers have breast cancer do fine, but we do need to recognize that some children have a particularly hard time with the reality of their mother's illness and are scared and worried. It is hard to know if these children are affected because their mother's experience was especially difficult (if, for example, her chemotherapy required her to spend weeks in the hospital) or because of their own personalities and coping styles. If you had to be away from your children for long periods of time or if your own physical or emotional trauma was clearly visible to them, they may be having a harder time recovering. As you think about your children and their adjustment to your diagnosis, there are some things to watch out for:

- Difficulties in school (academic, social, or behavioral)
- Behavioral problems at home
- Regressive behavior (e.g., thumb-sucking, bed-wetting, tantrums)
- Major changes in appetite
- Difficulties in sleeping or nightmares

- Major changes in behavior, such as becoming very timid or very aggressive
- Anxiety, either diffuse or focused on specific things
- Clinging to you or rejecting you

It can be hard to know what warrants worry and what does not. Teenagers, for example, always reject their parents, so how do you know whether their behavior is normal or evidence of a problem? My general suggestion is to trust your gut. You know your child better than anyone else does, and if you think he has a problem, you need to take care of him. If you observe any of these behaviors or if you simply feel worried about your child, do not hesitate to make an appointment with a child therapist. Choose carefully. Just as you yourself would want a therapist who is familiar with the issues facing cancer patients, you want your child's therapist to have experience working with children who are coping with parental illness. You can begin the search by speaking with your pediatrician, the school guidance counselor, or your own doctors or therapist. Taking your child to a therapist is not a sign of poor parenting or of actual trouble. It is simply an important way to prevent more-serious problems later on and to reassure your child that you will always respect and care for him or her.

As they get older, daughters are going to be worried about the impact of your breast cancer diagnosis on their own health. If other women in your family have had breast or ovarian cancer, and especially if you have been tested and found to carry one of the breast cancer genes (see Chapter 15), this is a valid concern. In such a case, you may want to suggest that your daughter read this chapter herself. If you do not have the positive genes, you can reassure your daughters that their risk of developing breast cancer is very minimally affected if your cancer developed after menopause, and that the risk is not seriously increased even if your diagnosis came before. You can also speak with your doctor about these risks, and, with his or her okay, invite your daughter to accompany you to that conversation.

Nonetheless, while these measures are useful, the truth is that words and reassurances don't help much with your own fears for them. The awareness that we may possibly, even very minimally, have contributed to our daughters' later development of breast cancer can be overwhelming. Try to remember that progress in early detection continues to be made and that it is probable that much better screening tests will be available in the future. Some doctors and scientists even talk about breast cancer prevention; that may be a real possibility by the time your daughters are adult women. At the very least, they will have a heightened awareness of this disease. They will do breast self-examinations, they will start getting mammograms in their thirties, and they will tell all their doctors about their family history. This vigilance will serve them well.

And the ultimate worry, of course, is your ongoing sadness and fear about the possibility of leaving your children. Betsy Lehman, a woman with breast cancer whom I loved and whose death was caused by a medication error during her bone-marrow transplant, spoke eloquently of this grief. She was often quite ill in the days following her chemotherapy treatments, and she described lying upstairs in bed and listening to the sounds of her family in the kitchen. "I lie there and I hear Bob talking to the girls and the clinking of dishes and their laughter. Instead of being glad that he is doing so well with them, all I can think is, *Is this how it will be after I die?*"

For women with breast cancer whose own mothers died of the disease sometime during their childhood, the burden of living on both sides of the equation is staggering. They know all too well the impact on a child of her mother's death. Reminders about advances in breast cancer treatment and much-improved survival rates do little to ameliorate their fear. Judith A. Ross, a writer in her forties, contributed an essay about this fear to our annual collection of survivors' writings:

> I dreamed I was with my mother last night. In the dream, I was calling for her in my sleep and she was lying next to me on the bed saying, "I'm right here," and I kept thinking "No, you're not, you're dead." And I woke up wishing that in the dream, at least, I could have believed her, and that the safety net that was ripped out from under me the year I turned sixteen, the year she was diagnosed with cancer, was still there.
>
> Eventually, though, I learned to trust life again and through my twenties and thirties, I actually thought I would live happily ever after. The pall of hereditary cancer hung over me but I hoped I could evade it. Now that it's happened, I am relieved that the suspense is over. But the world is once again a dangerous place. I'm like my nine-year-old son, full of fears and worries, and sometimes I'm a real pill. Unlike him, a trip outside to

look at the stars won't help with the kind of darkness I fear. I can't just pull down the shades to keep the bad guys away. No one can promise me perfect health.

I don't want my family to suffer because I am angry. It's not that I'm abusing anyone, but once in a while our home becomes a very tense place. I know there are no perfect wives or mothers, but every mistake I make feels as though it has lifelong consequences because I no longer assume that my life will be long. I wonder a lot about my boys. What memories of me will they keep?

Maybe they will remember me lying beside them saying, "I'm right here."

Still, although you could not protect your children from the reality of your cancer diagnosis, you can, to a greater or lesser degree, protect them from your ongoing worry about the future. Your younger children will not be aware, and should not be, of the stealth of breast cancer and the frightening reality that it can recur even years after the original diagnosis. Nor is there any reason to force this information onto your older children, although it is likely that they will have a better understanding of cancer's potential to recur. If you wish, with late-adolescent and young-adult children, you can certainly speak of your worry that it someday may come back and can share your fears and worries to the extent that you wish. But always remember that even adult children want desperately to believe that you have been cured. It is in no way helpful to them to dwell on the possibility of recurrence. This worry belongs to you and to your husband.

The truth is that the only things that will really help

your aching heart are luck and the safe passage of time. In the meantime, there are a few practicalities that can alleviate some of your concrete worries. You must have a will and you should prepare a careful financial plan. All parents should have these safeguards in place, but many do not. For you, there are no more excuses. Identical to my advice to women contemplating pregnancy after breast cancer, this is the time for you and your husband to have a thoughtful discussion about what would happen to your children should you both die. While you are now worried that you might die of breast cancer, you need to remember that people die of many other causes, too. As a responsible parent, you have to consider this terrible possibility. Talk with the family members, ideally, or the close friends whom you would want to raise your children. Confer with a capable lawyer so that the legal work is correctly done. Try to arrange your estate so that the guardians of your children will have adequate funds for their needs and education. And then try very hard to put these particular worries aside and get on with your life.

Some women decide to keep a scrapbook or journal for each child. These will be a treasure for them even if you live to a ripe old age. Your children, especially your young children, will never really know you as you are right now, so give them your current self in writing. It may also help you put aside your breast cancer and revalue what matters most; making an ongoing journal of moments with your children and family will help you pay closer attention to them. The goal is not to create diaries or journals of your deepest feelings but to capture moments in time, especially those that you are sharing with your children now. These suggestions are certainly not meant to be preparations for dying; rather, they are suggestions for living well. Saving your past and savoring your present will enrich your life as well as theirs.

12

Parents

When I was eight months pregnant with my second child, my mother was diagnosed with breast cancer. I was sitting next to her when her surgeon gave her the news, and I remember that the first thing she said to me was, "What have I done to *you*?" Nearly thirteen years later, when my surgeon gave me the same news, I was heartsick at the thought of having to tell her that her worst fear had come true. Given that my mother was in her sixties at the time of her diagnosis and no other women in our family have had either breast or ovarian cancer, it is unlikely that she passed a high-risk breast cancer gene on to me. But I knew that the facts of genetic susceptibility would have little meaning to her and that she would feel responsible and guilty.

She was then living in California with her second husband, and I waited a day to make the telephone call. First I needed to talk with my daughters, cry with my fiancé, and begin to assimilate the reality. As I write this, I am amazed that

I have no memory at all of the conversation that my mother and I must have had. I can remember every detail of telling my girls, my brothers, my friends, but I cannot remember a thing about telling my mother. That lapsed memory is powerful evidence of how painful our talk must have been.

My father had died of lung cancer fifteen years earlier. He was a nonsmoker, active, and healthy; then he was dead in six weeks. His acute illness and death had been our family's first experience with cancer, and when my mother was diagnosed two years later, it was hard for us to believe that she might do well. Fortunately, she was treated and seemingly cured, but she was certainly not prepared to have a daughter with breast cancer.

Your relationship with your parents, whatever its intensity and quality, is of singular importance in your life. Whenever I talk with a new patient, I ask about her parents. No matter how old we are, or even whether our parents are living, their influence and presence loom large in our lives.

Obviously, women who have lost a mother to breast cancer can be most powerfully affected emotionally by this tie. For many it will be almost impossible to believe that they themselves may be fine. The memories of their mother's illness and death haunt them. Very often, women in this situation say that they have actually been waiting for their own diagnosis, that there is even a certain perverse relief in its finally having happened. Many of these women are influenced by their mother's history in making their own treatment choices. That is, they may insist on the most aggressive possible treatment or, in an attempt to differentiate themselves, on something different from what their mother received. If this is your history, it is extremely important that you remind yourself that you are not your mother. Not only are the characteristics of your cancers likely to be dissimilar, but the available treatments are vastly different than they were twenty or thirty years ago.

Women whose mothers are breast cancer survivors have a somewhat easier time with this worry. They may be reassured by their mother's recovery and hope that their future will be similar. I have also known families in which the daughter's breast cancer preceded her mother's diagnosis. But, whatever the specifics, having several family members living with breast cancer is likely to be challenging to all concerned. Women cope in different ways. My own mother, a stoic and traditional lady, firmly believed in not dwelling on unpleasant things. As far as she was concerned, the minute that her treatment was over, the experience and the threat were over. During the months of her chemotherapy, when even she could not deny that something difficult was happening, she insisted on "pulling up my socks and putting my best face forward." She did not talk about the side effects and she certainly did not talk about her fear. I, on the other hand, make my living in the world of feelings. Affect and its communication are my currency. I needed and wanted to talk, and she could not bear to listen to me; she made her disapproval of my expression of my feelings very clear. Certainly this was due in part to genuine pain at my diagnosis, but it was also related to her belief that anger or tears or strong words are not proper behavior. One night several years later, I spoke with her about the next day's follow-up medical appointment, and I began to voice my anxiety.

She said in her old maternal, commanding voice, "Your cancer will not come back, and you need to stop worrying. Right now." End of discussion!

In times of trouble, all of us long for our parents, usually for our mothers. Still, for several weeks after I was diagnosed, I dreamed every night about my father. The details of each dream varied, but the theme was the same: being with him, being hugged by him, and feeling safe and protected. Those wonderful feelings stayed with me during the day and were some solace. It makes no difference how old we are or how old our parents are. It even makes little difference what kind of mother our mother has been. We yearn for ideal mothering, and the fantasy persists even if the experiences were otherwise. In my groups, the conversation when women speak of their mothers is often tender and intimate, and their longing for closeness and understanding is palpable.

Ronnie described these complicated feelings well: "When I was sick and in treatment, I came to realize that you are never too old to need a little mothering, especially when you are sick and afraid. But on a recent trip I realized that my mother, as good as she is, is not at all maternal. She really never has been and she was incapable of giving me a little motherly affection or care. I guess I still wish for more."

There are mothers and fathers who rise to this occasion splendidly. In fact, several of my patients have felt that their parents were much more nurturing during their cancer than they had ever been during their childhood—a second chance that sometimes enables parents and their adult daughters to forge an intimacy that otherwise would never have happened. But this is, of course, an ideal outcome; it is more likely that your parents have behaved during this crisis as they have during other crises in your life. Supportive parents stay supportive, and uninvolved parents stay distant. If your parents have disappointed you, the hurt may feel even greater now. At a time of vulnerability and need, it is very hard to accept that your parents, yet again, could not give you what you needed.

The importance of your relationship with your parents, your history with them, and their own needs and lives are relevant to your recovery in several ways. The impact of your diagnosis on them cannot be overestimated. No matter how old you are or how independent you are, you are still their daughter, their baby. Just as you try to protect and shelter your children from harm, they have wished to protect you. I have heard many elderly parents say, "It should have been me. Why couldn't it have been me? Why did this happen to her?" Depending on how old they are, your parents may also have a different view of breast cancer than your generation. Some will remember when it was "the C word," never to be mentioned in public, or they recall the years when women who were diagnosed with breast cancer told no one, were probably treated only with a radical mastectomy, and all too often died. They are very frightened by your diagnosis and may either have a hard time believing that you will be fine or, on the contrary, may be unable to admit that you might not be fine because that possibility is too painful to contemplate. They may want to know all the details of your diagnosis and treatment or they may want to know nothing.

A particularly poignant situation arises when one has living but very ill or demented parents. This is always a nightmare, but at a time of crisis it becomes even worse. Even though I strongly believe that honesty is almost always the best policy, these can be situations when *almost* is the important word. Some women decide not to tell a very frail parent about their breast cancer and are able, usually because of distance, to hold the secret. Occasionally, when treatment is over, this decision is reversed because it seems easier and less upsetting to tell when the crisis is past. More often, the secret is never shared, and there is relief in not having traumatized an elderly, fragile parent. You know your parents and your family situation best, but think very carefully about your reasons if you have chosen to keep the fact of your cancer from your parents.

Many middle-aged women find themselves taking care both of their children and of their aging parents. If you have had ongoing responsibilities for your parents' care, your illness has probably caused many problems. You will have had to work out other arrangements at a time when you were struggling to manage the logistics of your own life. If you have siblings, you needed to negotiate and rearrange the division of labor. Changes like these come at a cost, and you are now facing the consequences.

Some women described very difficult struggles with their parents or their siblings during their months of treatment. Elderly people frequently become self-involved and anxious; change is hard and frightening for them, so your parents may have seemed unable to understand or appreciate what was happening in your life that made you less available to them. They might have been very empathetic about your illness at one moment and at the next were complaining that you could not take them marketing. Hopefully, these disagreements are now past, but even if you were able to make some kind of accommodation to one another, there can be lingering hurt feelings on both sides that affect your relationship now.

Kathleen was a single woman in her early forties who came to speak with me some months after the completion of her treatment. She was a business consultant who had lived and worked in San Francisco, but because of a number of family problems she had decided to return to Boston. Kathleen moved into her own apartment and began to focus on creating a life for herself. Then her father died and she was diagnosed with breast cancer.

Hers was a high-risk breast cancer and she opted for very aggressive chemotherapy. Often, she had to stay in her mother's new apartment in a retirement community to recover after her treatments and she found the experience unnerving. "I felt weak and sick and terrible, but even in that condition it was weird to have all these healthy old ladies taking care of me." When she was finally well enough to return to her own home, she found that all the old family assumptions had resumed. It was expected that she would assist her elderly relatives as needed, help manage the family business, and be generally available as called upon. As she said plaintively, "Now that I am hoping just to live and have a life, I keep wondering whose life is this anyway?"

It is unimaginably painful for your parents to acknowledge the possibility that they might outlive you, and it is equally painful for you to contemplate this. However, just as you must plan for your own children, you must think about your parents' needs. Ideally, they have made plans for their later years and are not relying on you for care or support, but if this is not the case, you need to think about other arrangements. If you cannot talk with your parents about this, you must talk with your siblings. If you are an only child or are the only one responsible for your parents, you should speak with an attorney or an estate planner. The last thing you need is worry about how your parents will manage if your health is compromised.

Assuming that you stay well and live long, this offers you an opportunity to evaluate your relationship with your parents and even to make some changes. You may be closer to or more distant from them than you were before your illness, and they may have surprised or disappointed you. But while you can't change them, you can change yourself. In thinking about your priorities and values, you may decide that being closer to your parents matters to you; it is also possible that you will sadly conclude that a different—a better—relationship is impossible. These relationships encompass a lifetime of history that cannot always be amended.

Still, the fact that your illness has forced you to contemplate your mortality guarantees that you will reminisce about your life as well as frame your hopes for your future. This is a chance to make peace with your feelings about your parents.

13

Friends

One of the more unpleasant surprises for most of us is the change in friendships that cancer brings. The first inkling of this probably came at the time of your diagnosis. Almost all women talk of the unexpected reactions of friends. Even longtime ones may have simply disappeared. Others whom you barely knew became close friends during the months of your treatment. Overall, help and support have probably not come from all the expected places but have come from some you did not expect. You may have made new friends with women whom you met in the waiting rooms, treatment areas, or support groups that you attended. Moreover, it is likely that changes like these will continue after your treatment is over.

It is well known that any life crisis results in the loss of some friends and the gain of others. We commonly hear from people going through divorce or separation that some of their married friends have stopped calling. After a death in the family, people often find that some so-called friends are no longer a presence in their lives. The likeliest explanation for these disappearances—a reason, and definitely not an excuse—is that your experience has so frightened or threatened them that their only way to protect themselves is to avoid contact altogether. If a person's own marriage is shaky, it can be too scary to be around someone who is going through a separation; a cancer diagnosis is no different from any other crisis in its power to threaten others' sense of security. Indeed, because cancer is so unpredictable, so seemingly random in its victims, and so uncertain in its outcomes, your diagnosis may be even more frightening.

The converse—and this, too, happens—is the unexpected appearance of people who are drawn to others' troubles. My patients often tell me that they hear from people they knew barely or not at all. A neighbor or a friend of a friend calls to express sympathy and ask questions. In general, interactions like these are unwelcome. They seem intrusive and peculiar; none of us likes the feeling that we are the object of pity or a ripe topic of gossip.

Just as some people vanished around the time of your diagnosis, you will find that some disappear now that your treatment is over. It can again be helpful to remind yourself that this behavior has much more to do with their needs than with you. It is a reality that we all have busy lives; some friends will feel that now that they have done their duty to you, they can resume their usual routines without needing to make time for calls or visits. It is also a reality that some people were present during your months of vulnerability because their ability to help you made them feel good.

Once you are more or less back to yourself, they feel less needed and so move on to someone else.

And sometimes we ourselves may be the problem; our friends just can't win. It can make us angry if they continue to call daily, asking in a worried voice, "How *are* you?" but hold back about their own lives and concerns "because they seem so minimal compared to what you are going through." We want to feel normal by now. On the other hand, if they act as though we are completely back to normal, almost as if the cancer never happened, this too makes us angry. It is a fine balance that we seek from them, and their task can seem impossible, because we want different things from them on different days.

Most people have the luxury of not knowing as much about cancer as you do. They may think that once the treatment is over, the cancer is gone. They may ask questions like, "How do they test you to be sure that the treatment worked?" or even "Are you cured?" They may not recognize the one reality that you cannot escape: the hard fact that no one can ever promise you that the cancer is completely gone, that you are cured, that you can live the rest of your life without worry. The truth is that most of your friends just won't "get it." Whether this results from their wish to believe that you are fine, their inability to tolerate uncertainty and sadness, or a failure to understand the nature of cancer is irrelevant. They simply cannot fully grasp what you are feeling now.

Beth, a business consultant in her early forties, had breast cancer twice. The first time was a tiny tumor that was discovered during surgery for breast reduction. She was treated then with a wide excision (lumpectomy) and radiation. Six years later, she was diagnosed with a brand-new primary breast cancer in her other breast. Although the tumor itself was not very different from the first one, standards of care had changed in the interval, and this time she was treated with surgery, radiation, and chemotherapy. Understandably, she feels especially vulnerable and uncertain about her future.

"I've had people practically yell at me if I voice any kind of sadness, doubt, or fear," Beth said. "When I told my very best friend that I was afraid that my treatment plan would not go well, she shouted into the phone, 'Beth! Don't you believe in God?' I've had several people confuse my being realistic about the facts of cancer and treatment with being pessimistic or 'not having a positive attitude.' What non-cancer people don't understand is that we patients do not have the luxury of ignoring or 'tuning out' scary or unpleasant information. We have to become informed about the disease, and we have to undergo treatment that can be frightening and potentially damaging to our healthy cells. We have no choice. We cannot run from this stuff. We have to make the huge effort to deal with this disease and everything that comes with it.

"Noncancer people want desperately to believe cancer is always controllable, that once someone is treated, the cancer is absolutely gone and will never return. Cancer patients know better. But if we try to explain or enlighten noncancer people, we are usually met with blank stares or told to stop stressing, so we don't bring our cancer back."

When you are recovering from cancer, it can be especially hard to maintain a thick skin against remarks like these. Your friends are feeling freer to make the kinds of comments they would ordinarily; in fact, they may also feel free to express what they have been thinking during your months of treatment. Some so-called friends may actually tell you that you are selfish, cynical, negative, angry, or "always down." To some extent, these charges may be true. You have certainly been struggling with feelings like these, and you recognize that they are a normal accompaniment to cancer. They will gradually diminish, but it is understandable to worry that you will lose friends along the way. The best advice is to continue to express your feelings honestly, whatever they are, and to continue to make your friends aware of the normal recovery process. But it also behooves you, difficult though this may be, to assume an interest in their activities and problems. Real friendships are reciprocal, and at some point you will need to be an active and equal partner in giving as well as receiving.

As women, we treasure our friends. We depend on them and encourage them to depend on us. Cancer may strain these ties, so part of the challenge of recovery is continuing to value those relationships that have been sustaining, to repair some that have not, and to identify those that we should let go. These last may be among the biggest losses cancer brings you. More than one of my patients has spoken of having a major fight with a close friend during the first six months after treatment ended, during which the friend exclaimed, "It is *always* all about you!"

The fact is that your recovery *is* all about you. You are not the person you were, and you are still working your way toward being the woman you will become. It takes all your physical and your emotional energy to regain a sense of trust in your body and in your place in the world. It is important to find a way to explain this to your friends while being appreciative and respectful of their needs.

This is a major reason that many women find participating in a breast cancer support group so helpful. The women in the group have all been through what you have and are struggling with the same issues, so they will understand exactly what you need and have endless tolerance for the dialogue. One of the primary ways that people come to terms with any trauma is by talking about it. We need to tell the story over and over; as it becomes real in the telling, we begin to manage it. As we continue to recount it, we start to heal. Friends will not want to listen to it as often as you need to talk. You have to find others who can hear you with their hearts. As one woman said of her group, "When all is said and done, we are left with each other."

A major source of tension or even conflict with your friends is likely to be the change in your perspective. When you are worried about dying, it is impossible to empathize with a botched remodeling job or the cost of a trip to Europe this year. On your better days, you will be sufficiently aware of this to try to listen or pretend to care. On your not-so-good days, you may be bursting with anger or sadness. Wouldn't it be wonderful to have your biggest worry be your child's acceptance at her first-choice college!

You will have to educate your friends about cancer. You will need to tell them that you are doing your best to feel safe and strong. If you can, share with a few close friends what you need most in this time of recovery. Explain that you become particularly anxious in the days before a doctor's appointment or an annual mammogram. Perhaps ask whether they will mark these events on their calendars too and call you more often at those times. You may want to ask one of them to accompany you to these appointments or meet you afterward for lunch. Just as you learned how to ask for help and how to say "yes, thank you" when it was offered during your treatment, you will need to do this now.

If some of your friendships prove not to be the right match for you anymore, accept this, too. We have all had the experience of finishing school or changing jobs or moving and losing contact over time with close friends from the previous life. Breast cancer is just as significant a life event as those transitions, perhaps even more so, and in its wake there will be changes in some of your relationships. Give yourself permission to move on. Remember with fondness and gratitude those people who were your friends at another time in your life, and accept that they are not your friends now.

Human beings are remarkably resilient; they have the ability to make something positive out of almost any experience. Your friendships will be part of this transformation. As one woman said to me, "Just for the sake of the friendships I have made through cancer, I would never go back. Look at all that I would be missing!" The change of perspective that cancer brings enables us to become even more appreciative of the people we love. This is a point when we review our lives and reconsider our values. One benefit of the cancer experience for me has been the motivation to reconnect with some old friends and the joy we have found in our rediscovery of one another.

The new cancer friends you make are likely to be in a very special part of your heart. No one will understand what has happened to you like a woman who has also been through it. You will laugh and cry together in a communion that is only possible for soul mates. You will share each other's fears and joys as though they were your own and recognize a bond, forged in fire and pain, that glimmers now with hope.

14

Professional Issues

For many of us, work is an enormously important part of our lives. It fills our days with routine and purpose, it pays the bills, and it often defines our sense of who we are and how we think of ourselves. Breast cancer has a major impact on our work, and by the time you are reading this book, you will have already made decisions about working during treatment and telling your colleagues about your cancer during the acute phase of your breast cancer experience. But it's not over. You now have to contend with how work fits into your current life, what the implications of your illness have been and may be for your professional future, and how best to manage this important part of your days.

As one of my patients said: "I experienced considerable emotional distress, fatigue, and self-doubt in the months that followed active treatment. My supervisor could not see the need for me to attend your support group meetings once treatment was over. She expected me to snap out of it and to be back to 'normal.' Yet this period was more challenging than the treatment period. In my case, low blood counts lowered my energy level and productivity. I found that I was working on weekends to finish what I had failed to complete during the week. For someone who had always pushed to do more than necessary, this change was devastating."

There are a number of concerns about professional and work-life issues that follow breast cancer. Many women find that perspectives regarding their professional lives change as they go through the breast cancer experience. They have decisions to make both about returning to work and about the work itself. If you have been away from work on disability or another form of leave, it is important to think carefully about the timing of your return. If at all possible, you want to avoid coming back too soon, lest you discover you need to take another leave or find yourself not fully able to do your job. As you consider going back to work or resuming a full-time schedule, think about both your physical and your emotional health. Think about the demands of your ordinary workday. Is your energy higher in the morning or in the afternoon? Can you manage the commute? Is there training that you need? Talk with your supervisor and with the human resources staff before you return to insure that everyone shares the same plans and expectations for your reentry.

If you have been away from your job for many months, you may have lost some of your self-confidence. You may work in a field where six months or a year away really makes a difference. It may help to attend seminars or workshops or to read the most current professional literature to help you refocus your thoughts and skills. You might also consider going into work one or two part-days before your official start date. This will give you a chance to talk to your colleagues, catch up on office news, and begin to again feel at home in your work world.

If you are looking for a new job, you also have to consider what to tell prospective employers about your health history. You do not have to mention your cancer diagnosis any more than you have to share other personal details about your life—for example, whether you are married, have children, or where you live. It is generally wiser not to offer the information about cancer during early interviews. After you have been offered a job, you may decide to disclose your situation. You will be needing some time off from work for medical appointments, and getting an early sense of how difficult or not that may be will help you decide about accepting the job. Make sure that you present yourself as now being in good health, and reinforce the fact that you fully expect to stay well and handle the responsibilities of the position.

During the interview process, do not concentrate first on questions about medical-insurance benefits. If you have not yet told the interviewer about your cancer, focusing on medical insurance may tip your hand prematurely. You will want to know about all employee benefits, and asking about the total package will give you other important information, too. Once you have accepted a position, you will need to be completely honest with any questions about your medical history on applications for insurance. Do not try to "fudge" an answer or you could end up with much more trouble on your hands. Some jobs require a preemployment physical examination, and you certainly can't hide your scars from a physician.

You will also have to decide how to update your résumé and "explain" the time you have been away from work. If you are specifically asked in an early interview about a period of absence from the workforce, you can respond with a general statement about needing time for family matters or business.

Returning to or continuing with work following treatment of a life-threatening illness is challenging. You are likely to find that some of your work relationships have changed, that it may be difficult to work the same long hours that you did prior to your diagnosis, or even that you wish that you were doing something entirely different. Before cancer, much of your life and your sense of self may have been primarily related to your work. Is this still true? Your job is not your life, and breast cancer makes this very clear indeed.

Much of this book has been focused on the changes in our priorities and perspectives that accompany the onset of breast cancer. Most of us do become increasingly clear about what and who are most important in our world. Work is a crucial part of life: recall Freud's saying that what matters most are love and work. While we work for financial reasons, many of us would choose to work even if money were not an issue. Just as you now have little patience with negative people or with obligations that bring no pleasure, you surely have less patience with an unsatisfying work life. As you contemplate how to structure your life after cancer, thinking about how and where and why you work is of great importance.

There are women who make enormous changes in their work following cancer. I have known some who quit long-time careers to pursue a dream, who reduced or changed their work hours to make time for a hobby or to go back to school, or who added new responsibilities to their jobs and felt more fulfilled. As is true in all aspects of your life now, the important thing is to ask yourself the questions worth asking. Do you like the work you do and the people with whom you spend your workdays? Do you feel appreciated and valued? Does your work allow for flexibility and personal growth? Are the financial or psychological rewards commensurate with how hard you have been working? All these can be reduced to a single query: Knowing as you now do that life is fragile and may be short, is this how you want or need to spend your time?

Ann described the complications and texture of her work in this way: "I was in the middle of interviewing for a job change when I was diagnosed. I received a job offer just as I was making treatment decisions. I realized that I needed to tell the hiring manager what was going on in my life and that it was not a good time to be making a job change. I was frank with him; I said that I anticipated I would need some time off and had no idea what else was coming. I was stunned when he told me that he used to be a minister and went on to say many comforting and supportive things; in fact, I think that he opened up and shared more of himself as a person than he would have otherwise. He also said that he would call me in a few months to see whether I was

ready to work then and suggested that I might want to begin on a part-time schedule.

"He called as promised, and I started working on the
same day that I started my radiation treatments.

"There is, however, a downside. Although overall I feel
as competent in work as ever, I am much less ambitious and
hard-driving now. My self-confidence, especially in terms
of my appearance, has diminished greatly. This causes me to
hold back and take fewer risks. I am quite sure my coworkers see me as considerably older and less intense than they
would have if I had not had cancer. It's disconcerting when
they open doors for me and don't call me by my first name."

Issues around self-confidence and self-esteem are common and often difficult to resolve, especially if you feel less
sharp mentally and less strong physically. "I have been in
tears lately with my intensifying difficulty in retrieving
'stuff' that is in my brain somewhere," Linda said. "It is frustrating, scary, and time-consuming to have to do the same
things over and over because I forget the obvious steps. The
worst was a recent conference call with ten people, mostly
physicians. I referred to one doctor as 'she,' forgetting that
she is 'he'; I think I recovered reasonably well since two
people started talking at once, but that was sheer luck." Experiences like this are very upsetting.

Another common irritation is to find yourself the office
"cancer magnet," the person your fellow workers come to
whenever they have a friend or relative who is diagnosed or
they hear something interesting on the news about cancer
treatment. If these incidents are upsetting, it will be up to
you to find ways to set appropriate boundaries with your
colleagues.

All these changes in work relationships, whether perceived or real, can be challenging. As is true with family and friends, your colleagues and your supervisor are eager to believe that your problems are over. Their patience for further time off for medical appointments may be limited. If you continued to work throughout your treatment, colleagues may now feel that you have had your share of a reduced schedule or workload and may press you hard to resume long days. Cathy commented: "I have been close to tears or have shed them at points for almost two weeks. I just finished my first week of full-time work, and I'm exhausted. I am so sick of telling everyone, 'I'm fine,' and hearing from them how 'good' I look when I don't feel fine at all. I am incredibly weak and out of shape and fat. Who wants to hear that? My hair is gray, I can't exercise without hurting myself, and I am worried about the credit-card bills I have racked up over the past months. Meanwhile, my colleagues just want me to work harder."

A second general area of work-related concerns has to do with issues involving employability and benefits, especially insurance, that may be affected by your medical history. Most of us acquire our medical coverage through our employers, and you may find that good medical benefits have greater value now than extra vacation days or even a slightly higher salary. It is crucial not to let your medical insurance lapse for any reason! While it is possible to buy new insurance under an individual policy if you have gone uninsured for a while, any new policy may be limited by preexisting-condition clauses or by other restrictions that might impinge on your health-care options. This situation is less dire in employer-offered medical insurance, because the Health

Insurance Portability and Accountability Act of 1996 (HIPAA) limited the use of preexisting-condition restrictions in such policies. Under the conditions of HIPAA, no employer with two or more current employees can deny any employee coverage because of health status or preexisting conditions. While there are some restrictions under HIPAA (for example, if you have been uninsured immediately prior to enrollment, a group policy can still impose a twelve-month waiting period before preexisting conditions are covered), it is an enormous help to individuals who have a history of cancer or other serious illness.

However, HIPAA does not apply to individual policies. If you do find yourself without insurance, therefore, the best way to get it is, of course, to take a job that includes medical-insurance coverage. Obviously this also applies to coverage under a spouse's or, in some states, a same-sex partner's employee benefits. If this is not possible, you do have some other options. Call your state insurance department and ask if there are annual open-enrollment periods when insurance companies are required to accept new clients. Ask, too, whether your state has a high-risk insurance pool for people who otherwise might be uninsurable. Also call the largest insurance companies operating in your state, including Blue Cross, and ask if they have an open-enrollment period. If you are self-employed or work in a very small business, you may also be able to buy medical insurance through your professional organization, the Better Business Bureau, or the local chamber of commerce. The bottom line is that you may have to be persistent and creative, but you *are* likely to find a way to buy medical insurance.

In addition to concerns about medical coverage, you will now find it very difficult and often impossible to purchase individual life or disability insurance. This is not the case when such policies are standard benefits in medium- or large-size businesses. If your employer offers an annual opportunity to increase the limits of your life insurance without a physical examination, take advantage of it. If you have insurance through your employer but you change jobs and your new employer does not provide this benefit, try hard to keep your current policies and convert them from group to individual coverage. If you leave a position for any reason other than disability, it is often possible to convert them without providing proof of your health or insurability. Make careful inquiries of the human resources department of your company and with the insurance company itself, checking and double-checking the answers. Then follow the directions *exactly;* you do not want to give the insurance company any excuse to terminate the policy. An attorney who works with many cancer patients suggests that anyone seeking new life insurance should be prepared to make multiple phone calls and should be very careful about disclosing any more personal information than is requested. Also be aware that, even if you do find a way to purchase life insurance, there is almost certain to be a two-year period that you must survive in order for the benefits to be paid.

Disability insurance may be even more important than life insurance. Even if you do not have children or other family members to whom you would like to leave an inheritance, it can be important to have a source of income if you should become ill or disabled and unable to work.

Disability insurance is a common employment benefit but one that you are unlikely to be able to purchase on your own after a cancer diagnosis. What seems especially unfortunate is the fact that it is even difficult, if not impossible, to purchase a disability policy that excludes disability related to cancer but would at least cover other situations.

Two major government disability programs are helpful to people who do not carry private or employer-provided disability. Social Security Disability (SSD) and Supplemental Security Income (SSI) are both managed by the Social Security Administration. You are entitled to SSD if (by its definition) you are considered to be disabled for a continuous period of a year or longer *and* if you have worked and paid into the Social Security system for a designated number of quarters; the number of required quarters depends on your age at the time you file for disability. SSI is means-based, so it is available only to people who have limited financial resources; it does not require a person to have been employed and to have paid into the system. To determine your eligibility for either program, as well as the amount you can expect to receive, contact your local Social Security office.

You may find that you are facing discrimination in the workplace and that your choices feel limited. Even though women often find that their workplace and their coworkers are an enormous source of support both during and after cancer, there can be exceptions to this, and many women worry about the security of their jobs and their professional futures. I recall a story that I heard from a woman who worked for one of the large consulting firms. Throughout her treatment, she continued working long hours, traveling and trying very hard to maintain her previous level of productivity. When she met with her boss for her annual review, he complimented her on her hard work and noted that she had done well in spite of the rigors of her treatment. But then he went on to say that she would not be receiving a raise or a bonus that year because "I know you can't quit." She was furious, and then even angrier when she realized that, at least for the moment, he was right. She did not have the energy to engage in a job search, and she was unsure how prospective employers would react to her recent cancer history.

Perhaps the single most important piece of legislation for people who have had cancer or other illnesses is the Americans with Disabilities Act of 1990 (ADA). This law upholds your right to work in spite of cancer and in spite of the possibility of your needing special arrangements such as flexible work hours. The ADA protects you from discrimination in hiring, promotions, and salary; entitles you to special accommodations, such as a change in work schedule to permit medical appointments; and includes standards pertaining to confidentiality and disclosure.

In January 2002, however, the Supreme Court ruled that the ADA need not be as broadly applied as had been assumed. In order to be considered disabled and to qualify for protection under the act, an individual must be limited in what are called activities of daily living (ADL), not merely in particular job functions. This ruling has specifically defined disability under the act as limitations in ADL—being unable to manage these daily needs such as dressing, bathing, or preparing food. The common example given is of carpal tunnel syndrome. A person with this condition cannot perform repetitive movements on an assembly line but is able to manage daily activities, so he or she cannot invoke the protection of the act. If you have questions about the ADA or about a particular situation that you are encountering, you can call the Equal Employment Opportunity Commission (800-669-4000) for direction.

Unfortunately, we all acknowledge that discrimination does sometimes happen and that it can be very difficult to prove. An employer can usually cite a reason other than cancer to explain a missed promotion or a decision to not offer a job. If you feel quite certain that you have been discriminated against—that decisions like these were based on your health history—you may want to consult with a lawyer. He may tell you that little or nothing can be done to change the matter, but he may also have strategic suggestions about how to talk with your employer in ways that might improve your situation.

The second important piece of legislation to be aware of is the Family and Medical Leave Act (FMLA). Although primarily intended to protect the right of individuals to take time away from work to care for a family member, it also protects your right to request a leave because your health requires it. This may be interpreted as a period of weeks away from work or as intermittent hours or half-days to keep medical appointments or to manage fatigue. You are eligible for such leave if you work for the federal or any state or local government or for any private employer with more than fifty employees, provided that you have worked for this employer for at least twelve months. If you are interested in using your rights under this act, you should speak with your human resources department. Again, it is possible you may need to consult with an attorney, but it is likely not to be necessary.

In summary, as in all other parts of your life, you may find you will have to pay more attention to aspects of your work life that did not really concern you before cancer. You will think carefully about your work itself and what it means to you, about how you spend your time on and away from the job, and even whether it is time to make a change in your professional commitments.

15

Breast Cancer Gene and Genetic Testing

Genetic testing for breast cancer risk is a hot and controversial topic. First, some basics: As we know, our bodies are composed of billions and billions of cells, each with a specific design and purpose. In every cell there are genes composed of DNA that contain the operational blueprint for the normal, healthy functioning of that particular cell. Genes are the fundamental units of heredity in all living things, and when there is an alteration, or mutation, of the gene, that cell's behavior will be impacted. These mutations, which can produce a positive or a negative change in the gene, sometimes occur when DNA copies itself in the reproduction process. This results in a change in the genetic code that is then passed down to all future generations.

In 1994 scientists first identified the BRCA1 gene, which is present in everyone and which, when working normally, is thought to be useful in suppressing the abnormal growth of breast cells—in effect inhibiting the formation of breast cancer. However, it was then discovered that mutations in the BRCA1 gene can stimulate such growth and are associated with genetic or familial breast cancer, as well as with ovarian cancer. These cancers often develop at a young age and in both breasts (bilaterally).

You have probably heard of the so-called "Jewish breast cancer gene," technically called 185delAG. It is so named because mutations in BRCA1 and in a second gene, BRCA2, are more common among Ashkenazi (Eastern European) Jews who have a family history of breast cancer. (These mutations have also been found in French Canadians and some other populations but have been less studied thus far.) It is likely that there are other genes that also play a role in the development of breast cancer, but they have not yet been identified.

All of this means, obviously, that genetic tests are now available that can identify the presence of mutations in BRCA1 and BRCA2, and the emotional impact of contemplating or having such tests has been brought home very vividly by some of the women with whom I work. Considering this option, making the decision to proceed with testing, and then waiting five or six weeks for the results is psychological torture, even though these are women who already had breast cancer and who were aware that they came from families with a strong history of the disease.

How prevalent is genetically based breast cancer? It is estimated that heredity is a factor in 5 to 10 percent of all women with breast cancer. This means, of course, that 90 to 95 percent of women with the disease do not have a genetic predisposition to it. It is also important to remember that having the mutated form of these genes—that is, testing positive for one or the other of them—does *not* mean with certainty that an individual woman will develop breast cancer. But by age seventy, the incidence in such women is 55 to 85 percent, depending upon the strength of the family history of the disease.

Conversely, not having an abnormal gene does not mean that a woman can be certain that she will not develop breast cancer. She will still carry the same risk as all women in this country: approximately one in eight over her lifetime. Women who come from families with a strong breast cancer history who themselves test negative for the genes often feel somewhat skeptical of these results. Susan Love, M.D., identifies a third group, one that falls between those with a strong history of hereditary breast cancer and those with no family history at all. This group she terms *polygenic*—women who have a family history of breast cancer that is not directly passed on from generation to generation via one dominant gene. These polygenic women may eventually benefit from the discovery of additional gene mutations that predispose them to developing breast cancer. Until then, they are thought to be at higher risk of developing breast cancer than the general population, although less at risk than women with BRCA1 or BRCA2 mutated genes.

For obvious reasons there is great anxiety about genetic predisposition to breast cancer, and when there is a family history of the disease, women worry not only about themselves but also about their daughters and other female relatives. There is particular concern in the Ashkenazi Jewish community, where the incidence of an altered or mutated BRCA1 or BRCA2 gene is 2.5 percent (20 out of every 800 people). This is significantly higher than the incidence in the general population, where the rate is approximately 0.1 percent, or 1 in every 800 people.

Because men, too, have BRCA1 and BRCA2 genes, they can be carriers of the mutations. Since the incidence of breast cancer in men is very low, the more important concern here is the possibility of passing the gene on to their children. The child of a parent who has a positive gene has a 50 percent risk of inheriting the mutation. There is also some evidence that mutations in the BRCA1 and BRCA2 genes increase a man's risk of developing prostate cancer, and mutations in the BRCA2 gene are associated with an increased risk of male breast cancer and of pancreatic cancer. The risks for men are important to understand because, if the woman carries the gene, her sons may be affected; and if both she and her husband/partner carry it, their children are at very high risk.

The dilemma of whether or not to test is a good example of the difficulties raised when advances in technology and scientific knowledge are not matched by thoughtful policies pertaining to the many moral, legal, social, and health issues involved. Who benefits from genetic testing? What are the implications of either a positive or a negative result? How will these results be used, and will those solutions turn out to be in the best interest of the individual?

Genetic testing for the breast cancer genes involves only a simple blood test. Once the blood is drawn, it is sent to a designated laboratory for testing and evaluation, and the results are usually available in five to six weeks. (If there is an unusual situation of great urgency, the tests can be completed more quickly.) The test is available at commercial laboratories and within medical centers. Medical centers provide pre- and post-test counseling as well as considerable information about the procedure and its implications, but many for-profit laboratories do not offer either counseling or information. It is possible, and perhaps probable, that such commercial testing will eventually become widespread and even be encouraged as a part of standard health-care screening for all women.

It is my strong belief, as well as the belief of many activist groups, that for-profit testing like this should be discouraged and that any woman who is considering testing should do so only within the context of a medical center's designated program. Even though the test itself is minimally invasive, the complexities and implications of its findings are significant and often confusing. No one should have to contend with hearing the results of this test by herself. In addition, the only one who should interpret the results or explain their implications is a person who has been specifically trained in the area of genetic-cancer risk assessment.

How can you begin to consider this decision? Women who should speak with their doctors about testing include those who have had premenopausal breast cancer and have at least one first- or second-degree relative (mother, daughter, sister, grandmother, aunt, cousin) who also had premenopausal breast cancer or ovarian cancer, *and* women who have several relatives who have had either breast or ovarian cancer. If you have had premenopausal breast cancer, your sister or mother or adult daughter may also consider having this conversation. Women of Ashkenazi Jewish descent who have a personal or family history of breast or ovarian cancer are also candidates for testing. And some women who do not fit any of these categories still opt for testing as one way of easing their worry.

If your medical oncologist or surgeon is not extremely familiar with breast cancer genetic testing, it would be wise to make an appointment with a breast cancer high-risk specialist. Doctors with a particular interest in genetic risk and assessment in breast cancer can be found at major medical centers and are available for one-time consultation. You can call the division of oncology or the breast cancer center at such medical centers and ask if a high-risk specialist is on staff.

Choosing to be tested can be a way of taking more control of a seemingly out-of-control situation. Women who opt for genetic testing are usually those who have strong family histories or particularly intense anxiety about their future health. If the test is negative, this becomes one concern that you can jettison. If the test were to come back positive, it would provide you with concrete information.

Since you are a woman who has already had breast cancer, the implications of a positive gene test are significant. It is not known whether carrying a mutation in the BRCA1 or BRCA2 gene affects the prognosis for your existing breast cancer, but a positive gene does substantially raise the likelihood of a second unrelated breast cancer. For a woman who has a positive gene and has already had one breast cancer, the lifetime risk of developing a second new breast cancer can be as high as 65 percent. Having bilateral mastectomies would lower this risk by 90 to 95 percent.

In November 2001, a Mayo Clinic study was published in the *Journal of the National Cancer Institute* that demonstrated that prophylactic bilateral mastectomies reduced the risk of future breast cancer by 89.5 percent to 100 percent in women who were known to be carriers of mutations in the BRCA1 and BRCA2 genes. This study followed twenty-six high-risk women, who had all had this surgery, for an average of 13.4 years. So far, not one of them has developed breast cancer. It was calculated that without the surgery six to nine would have developed it. Although this study had a small sample size, the results are considered significant and important. As more time passes and more women are followed, it seems likely to be even clearer that prophylactic mastectomies are a powerful strategy in cancer prevention for high-risk women.

A positive gene-test result would also suggest that you consider an oophorectomy, or removal of your ovaries, because the risk of developing ovarian cancer is 20 to 50 percent. If you have had an estrogen-receptor-positive (ER+) breast cancer, the removal of your ovaries will also reduce the risk of a possible recurrence of your known cancer. It is estimated that removing your ovaries might reduce by as much as 70 percent the risk of developing a second breast cancer. Nonetheless, you should be aware that having all this surgery will still not lower your risk to zero. It is impossible for a surgeon to completely remove every iota of breast tissue in mastectomies, and despite an oophorectomy, an ovarian-cancerlike disease can still develop in the cells that line the inner abdominal wall. The risks are very greatly reduced, as noted above, but it is still possible that you could develop breast or ovarian cancer.

This is where the importance of having genetic testing done within a medical center that includes pre- and post-test counseling becomes especially important. If you should test positive, it may be wise to have several appointments to fully discuss your options and concerns with a therapist. It is no small matter to have both breasts and your ovaries removed. In addition to the physical trauma of the surgeries, you will have to cope with significant psychological trauma. Only after very careful thought can you make such a decision. A key consideration is how much anxiety you can live with. You may already have considered this question in the context of decisions regarding treatment for your breast cancer, and you may have opted for either more- or less-aggressive treatment based on your own personality style and your capacity for living with uncertainty and anxiety. Your choices now are even more formidable.

For women who opt not to have bilateral mastectomies, other screening tests may be recommended in an attempt to identify cancer at an earlier stage. Annual mammograms will continue to be important, but other screening tools may also be considered. Studies are under way to evaluate the value of breast MRI and PET scans in the early detection of breast cancer. The bottom line is that none of these tests are 100 percent accurate and that at best they detect a cancer that is already there. Still, while they have no value in preventing a cancer from growing in the first place, they may find it at a very early stage.

Since these genes also raise the risk of ovarian cancer, it is likely that your doctor would recommend annual pelvic ultrasounds and blood tests to check for a protein called CA-125, a marker for ovarian cancer. There are promising results in clinical trials that identify other blood markers in early ovarian cancer; these tests should be available in a few years. Ask if these or other tests would be appropriate and available to you and if your doctor feels that they might be helpful.

Remember that you do not have to make a decision immediately upon receiving news of a positive gene test. It is not a medical emergency. Nothing has actually changed except that you now know something that was previously unknown. Some women find a bizarre comfort in having a reason for their breast cancer diagnosis. They say things like, "Well, now that I know I have the gene, I know why it happened." It is also possible to make decisions in stages. I have known many women, for example, who quickly proceeded with an oophorectomy but did not have bilateral mastectomies.

Linda, a forty-year-old mother of two, knew that she had a strong family history of breast and ovarian cancer and that her genetic test was likely to be positive. Still, when the results came back and she was indeed positive for both the BRCA1 and the BRCA2 genes, she was devastated. The anger she felt at the time of her initial diagnosis returned with a rush, and it took time before she could settle down to consider her options.

Linda found that her feelings about her choices changed over time. Since she was not planning to have any more children, it was a relatively easy decision to have her ovaries removed. However, the possibility of having bilateral mastectomies was daunting. When her husband's sister, who had also had breast cancer, tested positive, Linda felt that the implications for her own children were unbearable. The reality that there were genetic factors on both sides of her children's heritage was stunning. Her daughters were old enough to understand some of the implications for them but were too young to make any decisions based on their own cancer risk, and the burden that telling them would place on their young shoulders was unbearable.

Thus far, Linda has opted to stay informed about any new studies or data, to have careful and frequent follow-up (mammograms, ultrasounds, breast MRIs, and physical examinations), and to live with the anxiety of a possible second breast cancer. At this moment she believes it would be emotionally easier to lose both of her breasts in the context of a second cancer diagnosis than to do so beforehand by choice. She thinks that, because she has already lived through one breast cancer diagnosis and treatment, she could do so again if necessary. Most important, she is living this decision in an ongoing way. She continues to evaluate her choices, to realize that she is always free to change her mind, and to focus on trying to live as fully and deliberately as possible, though this often is difficult.

Many women who have had breast cancer worry about the possibility of a gene mutation in terms of its impact on others whom they love. As Linda's story indicated, one of the most terrible aspects of breast cancer is the concern that you have increased your daughters' chances of developing the disease or have passed the mutated gene to your son, who might in turn pass it to his children.

Because the "remedies" for a positive gene test are really not remedies (even the drastic surgeries do not *eliminate* the risk of cancer) and because a positive test does not definitively predict that any one woman will go on to develop cancer, it is controversial whether genetic testing is advisable for your daughters. A compromise position might be for you to proceed with the test. If you do not have the gene, you can stop worrying about them in this respect. If you do test positive, they will have the option, as adults, to consider testing themselves. In fact, no medical center will test children or very young adults for the breast cancer gene mutations.

If your daughters are young now, it is likely that by the time they reach adulthood, more will be known about the risk reduction or even prevention of breast cancer. There is the real possibility of strategies that we cannot envision yet—possibly even gene therapy that replaces a defective BRCA1 or BRCA2 gene with a normal one. There is ongoing research in this area and reason to be cautiously optimistic about scientific progress.

Tamoxifen is also increasingly prescribed to high-risk women who have *not* had breast cancer. Usually these are women who have tested positive for mutations in the BRCA1 or BRCA2 gene and who are unwilling to act on the more-aggressive recommendation of bilateral prophylactic mastectomies. We now know that tamoxifen is most helpful for women who carry the BRCA2 gene and not the BRCA1. A study presented at the 2000 American Society of Clinical Oncology (ASCO) meeting examined thirteen thousand women at high risk for breast cancer who had been given either tamoxifen or a placebo. This study, known as the Breast Cancer Prevention Trial, found that tamoxifen reduced the incidence of breast cancer in some women. There are ongoing national trials for high-risk women who have not had breast cancer to further evaluate the effectiveness of tamoxifen. Your sisters, mother, or daughters might be interested in discussing these trials with their doctor. Obviously, this is a highly personal and difficult decision. Taking a powerful drug to treat a known breast cancer is quite different from opting to take it in hopes of preventing a future breast cancer. There are always risks as well as benefits to be weighed.

In summary, what does a positive BRCA1 or BRCA2 test result mean? Given that you have already had breast cancer, your doctor will spell out its implications for you and your future health. For women who have not had breast or ovarian cancer, a positive result means only that they have inherited the mutated gene and are at increased risk of developing either illness. But in both these situations it is important to remember that men and women who have the gene, whether or not they ever develop cancer, can pass the mutation on to their children.

What does a negative BRCA1 or BRCA2 test result mean? Although it certainly feels more reassuring to receive a negative rather than a positive result, in some ways a negative answer is not necessarily helpful. First, it signifies only that you do not have one of the identified gene mutations that increase risk. Scientists widely assume that there are many other genes associated with the development of cancer; we just do not yet know how to find and identify them. (It is also possible, although not likely, that the test somehow missed the mutation and that the negative answer is truly a "false negative.") Most important, a negative gene test does not mean that the individual will never go on to develop breast cancer. Remember that 90 to 95 percent of all breast cancers are not related to either BRCA1 or BRCA2.

The National Breast Cancer Coalition (NBCC) and the National Alliance of Breast Cancer Organizations (NABCO) have developed helpful materials regarding many issues related to genetic testing. Information is also available from the National Cancer Institute (NCI) and the American Cancer Society (ACS). In the "Resources" section at the end of this book, there is information about how to reach these organizations. The bottom line is that genetic testing for gene mutations is neither a straightforward nor an easy decision. If you are considering proceeding with this testing, be sure that:

- You talk with a specialist in high-risk cancer assessment and screening.
- You proceed with testing only at a medical center that also provides pre- and post-test counseling.
- At a medical center, you may be offered the opportunity to enroll in research trials looking at the value of certain kinds of follow-up or tamoxifen treatment for high-risk women. You may hear about clinical trials that are open to your female relatives if you should test positive. Carefully consider any that you might enter, thinking both

about their value to you and their value to the knowledge base for other women.

- You recognize how emotionally stressful the testing will be and try to prepare yourself for the process.

- You think about what you will do if the test results are positive. Clearly, this will be preliminary; you cannot know with certainty what your decisions will be until and unless you are faced with the hard questions, but it is empowering to gather information and consider your treatment options. Especially if you think you might opt for mastectomy (or mastectomies if you have not already had one), this is a good time to learn about the different reconstruction options. If you do test positive, it will be a more psychologically stressful period later.

- You do not make this decision in the immediate aftermath of your breast cancer diagnosis and treatment. Let some time pass before you proceed.

- You recognize that there are exceptions to the rule above. If a woman with a suspect family history has chosen to have a mastectomy and reconstruction as treatment for a known breast cancer, she may want to know the result of gene testing at the time of her surgery. Knowing of a positive genetic test, she might opt for bilateral mastectomies (with or without reconstruction) at that time. A single operation means one surgery, one anesthesia, and one recovery. Some women have been appropriately angry that this option was not mentioned at the time of their surgery and treatment for a known breast cancer.

One of my patients who had tested positive for the BRCA1 gene struggled for more than a year with the

decision of whether to proceed with bilateral mastectomies. Since writing is one way that she approaches difficult things in life, and her written words often enable her to
understand and process her feelings, she wrote this poem.
She brought it to one of our sessions and asked me to return it to her later, after she had made a decision. She knew
that she would then need reminding of what she had en-
dured and how she had finally chosen to proceed. Since
these words were part of her process and her pain and because each decision is so highly personal, I won't tell you
what she eventually chose to do. I will say that the time and
energy she expended were invaluable and that she is content with her decision.

UNTITLED

By Laurie Beth Gass

Whatever I decided, I did the best I could.
I was not a coward.
I found a way to hold this knowledge inside
without my brains or my heart exploding.
I wasn't alone yet I felt great loneliness.
Having this knowledge sucked! It also gave me the
choice to lighten my load against cancer.
Whatever I decided, I did so using all my
capabilities.
I had the full support of my life partner to make
any choice I wanted.
Barbara and I are friends for the journey, whatever
that is.

I was surrounded by a circle of friends,
supporters, and cheerleaders saying
"GO LAURIE."
WHAT IF? WHAT IF?
I can't live what if and as if. I'm going to have to
just live.

16

The Hard Part

Without question, the most anguishing part of having breast cancer is the immutable fact that this is a life-threatening illness. Although advances in early detection and treatment have improved both disease-free survival times and overall survival, far too many women still die of breast cancer. It is the second-largest cancer killer of women (after lung cancer) and the number-one cause of cancer deaths among women aged forty to fifty-five. In the United States, a woman dies of breast cancer every thirteen minutes.

It is impossible to minimize these realities. Because all of us face the possibility of a recurrence, this may be an especially difficult chapter to read. Following the diagnosis of cancer, a stricken individual almost always feels that she will die of the illness. As Carol said, "Those of us who have had cancer have been to the end of the precipice, looked down, faced the fear of falling, and have returned. Those people who haven't had cancer don't know that you don't have to fall when you are at the edge." Even today, there often seems to be a generation gap, with older people more likely to believe that a cancer diagnosis is inevitably a death sentence. Fortunately, this is often not true, but it can sometimes be hard to remember that. The heart-stopping fear usually diminishes over time, and you probably have long stretches now when you are able to feel quite hopeful about your future. How optimistic you can be is related to several things: your own temperament and coping style, the specific details and therefore the statistics that accompany your particular cancer, and how long it has been since you were diagnosed. Time helps. Luck helps more. Even women who have found ways to decrease their fears and to live their lives without undue anxiety may fall into unexpected rabbit holes of terror. All it takes is to come upon an obituary of someone your age who just died of breast cancer or to learn that someone you knew when you were both in treatment has had a recurrence or even died of her illness. Birthdays, anniversaries, holidays, and other marker events are also points when such feelings may intensify. Being prepared won't always keep them at bay, but knowing that these feelings may reappear unexpectedly can help you feel slightly more in control.

To some extent, surviving breast cancer seems to be a crapshoot. Of course there are innumerable studies and statistics to suggest that one or another woman is more or less likely to stay well. We all know that a smaller primary tumor is better than a larger one, that negative lymph nodes are better than positive ones, and that certain pathological features of the cancer cells are more or less worrisome. I also know that some women who had tiny primary tumors and negative lymph nodes have gone on to die of their disease, while others who had many positive lymph nodes and a much more serious initial presentation have stayed well. The truth is that you cannot know on which side of the statistics you reside.

Scientists and physicians are working hard worldwide to improve our current treatments and to someday find a cure. Many millions of dollars and countless hours are devoted to these efforts, and we all pray for their success. In the meantime, we can be grateful for the real progress that has been made.

Some women want as much information about their prognosis as possible; they may search the Internet and library for data that seem to apply to their situation. Others want to know as little as possible and try to focus on the present and their hope for the future. You know best what is right for you. If information helps you feel more in control, you should search for it. If you would prefer to not know specific data, that's fine, too.

Whatever your coping style, it is very important to remember that no statistic is predictive about any individual's life. Statistics are numbers gained from the study of large pools of people. They never speak directly to one woman. The survival statistic for each of us is either 100 percent or 0 percent. Remember, too, that any published data are already somewhat outdated. Clinical trials that are in process require years to produce information. For example, in comparing one adjuvant treatment to another, researchers must wait at least five—and probably ten—years after the last participant's treatment is completed before useful information is available. Sooner than that, they can know whether one treatment is more likely to extend the disease-free survival time (the length of time between diagnosis and a first recurrence), but more time must pass before they know whether that same treatment will indeed result in more women being alive and completely well after ten years.

One of the more frightening facts about breast cancer is that it can recur at any time. For many cancers, safely passing the five-year mark means that a person is almost certainly cured. For breast cancer, there is no such safe marker. The majority of breast cancer recurrences are diagnosed within the first five years, so once you have passed that anniversary of your diagnosis, you can breathe a half-sigh of relief. However, breast cancer can recur seven or ten or fifteen or even more years later. Oncologists wonder whether the future will produce more late recurrences because of the success of current adjuvant chemotherapies and hormonal therapies—that is, the possibility that these treatments will have delayed but not prevented recurrence in some women. When we look at graphs of survival, the curves definitely improve after the first few years, but the slopes never descend to zero.

There are two general kinds of breast cancer recurrences, and it is important to understand the difference. Sometimes the cancer returns in the same breast where it started; this is called a local recurrence, not a distant metastasis. Any recurrence that is outside of the breast is metastatic disease. A local recurrence often requires additional treatment only to the breast. If that breast has already received radiation, it cannot be radiated again. Very occasionally a woman who had a tiny original tumor may have had only a wide excision, no radiation. In her case, radiation would now be an option. For anyone else, the choice of local treatment is limited to a mastectomy. Reconstruction possibilities may also be more limited because of the tissue changes caused by earlier radiation therapy. Previously radiated tissue does not stretch or heal in completely normal ways, and reconstruction using an expander and implants may not be possible.

A recurrence in the skin of the chest wall can happen to women who have had a mastectomy. A mastectomy can remove only about 95 percent of the breast tissue; a recurrence can occur in the residual breast tissue that is usually located in the axilla (under the arm). This remaining breast tissue is different from the tissue containing axillary lymph nodes; a recurrence in an axillary lymph node is a slightly different situation. In the case of a recurrence on the skin of the chest wall after mastectomy, the treatment and prognosis is similar to that of a distant metastasis.

Women who have previously had mastectomies and who experience a limited chest-wall recurrence may have surgery to remove the nodules and then radiation to that area. If the chest-area recurrence is more diffuse, the local treatment may be radiation alone. These are decisions that must be made on an individual basis with your doctors. All in all, local recurrences (contained within the breast) are considered to be treatable and potentially curable. Just because cancer has returned in the breast does not mean that it has necessarily spread elsewhere in the body.

Further treatment for a local recurrence depends on your doctor's assessment of the risk of metastatic disease. Much like the careful physical workup done at the time of first diagnosis, your doctors will schedule X rays and CAT scans to find out if the cancer has also spread elsewhere. Even if those staging tests (scans, X rays, or MRIs) were negative, careful consideration would be given to the pathological features of the tumor. If the tumor has some aggressive features, it is possible that systemic treatment would be prescribed. This could include chemotherapy or hormone therapy or both. Unlike the situation with the initial breast cancer, there is no firm evidence that adding these treatments to mastectomy helps prevent additional recurrences.

It is important to make the distinction here between a local recurrence in the breast or skin of the chest wall and the development of an entirely new breast cancer (a second or new primary). A pathologist can differentiate between two cancers by comparing cells from each; it usually will be clear whether a tumor is a recurrence of the first cancer or a new one. We know that women who have already had one breast cancer are at higher risk of developing a second, unrelated breast cancer. If this happens, the second cancer is treated independently of the first. Unfortunately, that means you may have to go through the entire treatment experience all over again: surgery, radiation, and hormone or chemotherapy. (The choice of chemotherapy may be affected by the previous chemotherapy, because there are lifetime limits to how much of certain drugs one woman can safely receive.)

Unfortunately, I have known a number of women who developed a second breast cancer; it is obviously a traumatic and horrible experience. However, while this is not in any way intended to suggest that the diagnosis of a second breast cancer is easy to cope with, these women do tend to find some parts of the experience slightly less difficult than the first time. They already know and trust their doctors; they understand the treatment options; they are familiar with the landscape of cancer care. More importantly, they have been through this once and know that they can do it again. Finally, the prognosis of a second breast cancer is independent of the first; this may be less frightening than the realization that the treatment for the earlier cancer was not entirely successful.

The second and even more upsetting kind of breast cancer recurrence is a metastasis to another part of the body. Metastatic breast cancer most commonly develops in the lungs, liver, bone, lymph nodes at the base of the neck, or brain. Breast cancer that spreads (metastasizes) elsewhere in the body is still breast cancer—that is, breast cancer cells that spread to the lung, for example, are breast cancer metastases, not lung cancer. The term *metastatic breast cancer* is correct no matter where in the body the breast cancer cells may spread. If breast cancer cells are found to have spread somewhere in the body outside the breast, they are also assumed to be present elsewhere—even if they are too minute to be detected by scans or X rays. Single or small numbers of cells are too tiny to be seen. The systemic treatment that you have already undergone, whether chemotherapy or hormone therapy, was designed to eradicate any remaining cancer cells, wherever in your body they may have spread. Metastatic breast cancer results from the failure of the systemic treatments applied at the time of initial diagnosis to eradicate all such cells. Metastatic breast cancer is always treated systemically, and while it is very rarely curable, it is almost always treatable.

Many women can now live, and live well, for some years—occasionally for many—following this diagnosis. In the early years of my practice, I remember encouraging women in this situation that new advances were being made and that something helpful might soon be found. This was not untrue but it was something of a stretch. The same thing can more realistically be said today, for we recognize that a great many treatments for metastatic breast cancer are available that did not exist even a few years ago. Women who are living with metastatic breast cancer are living with permanent treatment, which will last for the rest of their lives. The general plan is the use of serial treatments; each one is used as long as it is helpful in controlling or reducing the cancer. Because breast cancer cells eventually become resistant to a particular treatment and stop responding, the treatment is then changed to a different one in the hope that it will be effective for many months.

Carol is a fifty-year-old artist who is living with metastatic breast cancer. She said: "This cancer thing is quite the experience. I was petrified of a recurrence, yet once it came, there was some sort of relief, as screwy as that sounds. I didn't have to worry about it anymore. Now I have to contain the disease, and that sometimes presents lots of complications. But I just went to Italy for a month and had a wonderful trip. I hope to go again.

"The long and short of it is that this disease has made me so thankful to be alive. We are all on the verge of passing from this planet at any split second, so all we ever have is this moment. It is our choice how to spend this moment, in fear or in joy. We forget how bad it can get. Last week I got a glimpse of the possibility that I might be leaving this planet sooner rather than later. I am delighted to say that I think I have a reprieve. Concentrate on your blessings."

Fear of recurrence and the realities of metastatic breast cancer haunt us all. They haunt our doctors, too. One medical oncologist, a dear friend, wept as she told me the news of a mutual patient's recurrence. "I feel so helpless," she said. I say to all my patients: "Let me take care of you. Do what I say, all the horrible things, and it will keep you safe. But of course we both know that there are no guarantees." The shared knowing that there are no guarantees is one of the reasons that we often feel especially close to our oncologists. Unlike most other doctors, our oncologists are important parts of our lives for all of our lives. Together we think and talk about both life and death; together we focus our hopes on life.

How do we manage to go on, given this fear? Learning to live with the sword of Damocles over us without letting anxiety and sadness paralyze us is the real challenge of life after breast cancer. The days will be rare that you don't give your death at least a brief thought. Barbara describes this as "not really frightening; it's more that the thought of my death has become a constant presence, something I just know is there." We gradually learn to live life on parallel tracks of hope and dire possibility. We find that each important decision is marked by a two-angle lens—there is the maybe-I-will-live-for-years view and the maybe-my-life-will-be-short one. Every such decision, every relationship, every plan must be forced through that double filter. Actually, I have found this dual view to be remarkably clarifying. It has become very easy to recognize what is important and what is the right choice.

Continuing on becomes above all else a search for sustenance and for meaning. Although we are living with what sometimes seems unbearable, it is that very burden that also gives light to our days. We are never again allowed to forget that life is fragile and fleeting and that it is our relationships that are the most important. We wrestle with life's great themes. Once we have been forced to recognize the omnipresent nature of endings and of loss, we have the choice of either retreating to denial and pretending not to notice or we can stand up straight, put our shoulders back, and face it. In staring down that tiger, we learn how to live. As Audre Lorde, a self-described black lesbian poet warrior who eventually died of breast cancer, said, "When I use my strength in the service of my vision, it becomes less and less important whether I am afraid."

The truth is that we are all afraid sometimes. Another part of that truth is that we find ways, often in community, to support one another and to face the fear. I facilitate a weekly group for women who have metastatic breast cancer, and I am regularly awed by their courage and their grace in accepting me as an equal partner in the journey.

Being with them helps me to imagine that I, too, can live with this challenge if it comes to me. There is deep comfort in this. As the women in this group often say, we learn from one another that there are worse things than death, and we learn how to meet death when we must.

Sometimes it is necessary and helpful to look directly at the fear and the possibilities. Pretending that they do not exist is rarely a useful strategy. This is not to say that it is necessary to dwell on them, but it is often helpful to think about them enough to become able to put them aside. Fears left unacknowledged are the proverbial elephant under the rug; you will end up tripping over them when you least expect it. It is not morbid or pessimistic or neurotic to think about your cancer returning. All of us have those moments, and the task is to learn somehow to get beyond the fear. As Amelia Earhart said, "Courage is the price that life exacts for granting peace."

When I talk with my patients about their fears, I suggest that we name them. Rather than worrying vaguely about "what if it comes back?" it can eventually be helpful to be more specific about them. What worries you most? Pain? Leaving your children, your spouse, or your family? Do you think about being a burden to your family? Do you worry about who will take care of you? Do you wonder whether you will be able to stay home or if you may need to be in a care facility of some kind? Do you then worry about what kind of facility this may be? What are you more afraid of: the process of dying or being dead?

Since the loss of control is one of the things that may upset us most, thinking about the particulars and imagining how you would handle them returns some control to you. I have known women who were reassured by learning about hospice services in their communities. I have even known a few women who were comforted by a visit to their local funeral home to make their own arrangements. If pain is what you fear most, your doctor can help you learn more about the excellent pain-management drugs and techniques that are available.

The most extreme example of such concerns is, for some women, the consideration of physician-assisted suicide. This is a much-discussed topic, and great controversy surrounds it. There are intense ethical, legal, and religious issues involved. It has been my experience that most people who are diagnosed with cancer at least think about suicide at one time or another. Statistically, fewer cancer patients commit suicide than people in the general population. However, most of my patients *have* talked about suicide, and especially about issues having to do with control, with pain, and with choice. What they usually are seeking is the belief that they can continue to be in control of their lives, and the reassurance that there is an "out" if they ever need it. Knowing that it may be possible usually neutralizes the issue. If you should want to, this is a conversation that you could have at some point with your doctor and/or with your husband or other adult family members.

Thinking and talking about the possibility of your cancer coming back or about your death does not make it more likely. Most of us are subject to the kind of magical thinking that makes us fear that saying something aloud makes it more real. This is simply not so. To the contrary, you are more likely to feel relieved and soothed after these very difficult conversations. Facing the tiger, saying the unthinkable, bearing the unbearable will help you put those fears in a better perspective.

17

Getting Support

Just as no woman should have to go through breast cancer treatment alone, no one should have to contend with the weeks and months after treatment by herself. A normal reaction to this experience is a sense of isolation or, at the least, feeling different from others. We all experience some degree of depression or anger or anxiety or discouragement in the months following treatment. While time will help, there are ways to identify and use support to accelerate the recovery process. What works best for one woman may be entirely wrong for someone else, but be reassured that there are many ways to build an individualized and effective support network. The goal of this chapter is to help you think about what you need and want most and where to find it.

There is no question about the value of social support for people with cancer. Looking at both their physical and psychological coping and recovery, study after study has found that those people who have multiple sources of support do better than those who are more isolated. The familiar song is right on track: "People who need people are the luckiest people in the world." People who care about us and for whom we care are an endlessly renewable resource.

Earlier chapters talked at length about relationships with your husband or partner, your children, your parents and extended family, your friends. They all have an important place in your heart and in your life and will contribute to your growing sense of well-being. As discussed earlier, you may have to educate some of them about what you are feeling and what you seek from them—and do not be surprised if you need to tell them more than once.

Be as specific as possible when you talk with them about the ways in which they can help you. It may be that you want their reassurance that you will be fine, or you may find such words infuriating. Perhaps you want them to distract you when you are feeling sad or scared, to insist that you come along to the movies even if you don't feel like going, and to reach out to you in reliable and consistent ways. On the other hand, the extra attention may feel smothering, as if their frequent calls or visits mean that they believe you won't be around much longer. You need first to be clear inside yourself about what you want from the important people in your life. They can't know and they are likely to make mistakes if they are left to their own imaginings. Figure it out and tell them clearly. And remember to thank them when they do what you have asked of them!

One of my patients told me a lovely story about the importance of relationships. She was playing tennis three months after completing her treatment. During a break in the game, she noticed two aged women who had stopped to watch the play. As they walked away from the tennis courts, their arms interlocked, one turned and said to the other, "Rachel, we made it through another winter." Sue said she had to pinch herself to realize that they were speaking to each other, not to her. Life after breast cancer is moving toward spring. It is the "arms interlocked" quality of our relationships that helps us through the winters and toward the more gentle warm air.

As will be discussed in the next chapter, many people are enormously helped and comforted by their faith. It may be that speaking with your minister, priest, or rabbi will be reassuring as you move through the months of recovery. Even if you are not an active member of a church or temple but now feel that such a relationship could be helpful, it is still possible to talk with a member of the clergy. Call one of the larger churches in your town and ask. There are also pastoral counselors who work at many hospitals and faith-based social-service agencies.

In thinking about what will be of help to you during this period of recovery, it is useful to remember other difficult times in your life. Strategies that worked then are likely to help now, too. For example, women who have previously used meditation or yoga or weekly massage during times of stress may find them valuable. Others who have participated in support groups focused on various life problems—whether they are programs like AA or Al-Anon or groups for people trying to stop smoking or live with rebellious adolescents—are often very early recruits to breast cancer groups. Having learned that such groups are helpful, they seek out similar programs during this new crisis.

Obviously the stresses associated with your diagnosis, treatment, and recovery differ from those associated with other life problems. The solutions will differ, too. While some life problems must be borne alone, breast cancer is not one of them. It is both my experience and my bias that participation in the community of women who have had breast cancer is extremely valuable for most women coping with this disease and its aftermath. For better or worse, the epidemic of breast cancer means that there are many women who are living through this experience with you. Joining with them in some way will help you better understand and manage your feelings. It is enormously relieving to recognize that these feelings are normal and shared by others.

There are several kinds of groups often available for women who have had breast cancer: psycho-educational or information groups, on-line chat rooms or support groups, self-help groups, professionally led support groups, stress-management groups, and one-time seminars or lectures devoted to specific topics. Psycho-educational or information groups are organized around issues and generally involve different expert speakers at each session. A typical series of such a group program might include biweekly meetings about psychological coping, fatigue, family relationships, future directions in breast cancer research, issues in the workplace, and complementary therapies. In a ninety-minute meeting, there might be a forty-five-minute lecture, a half-hour question-and-answer period, and some time for socializing. Sometimes the participants have an opportunity for input in planning the series, and sometimes the schedule is organized before the group is announced.

On-line chat rooms and support groups are newcomers to the field. The Internet can provide enormous amounts of information and support in the area of breast cancer. The major problem, as is true of researching any subject on-line, is that it is very difficult to assess the value and validity of what you find. This becomes especially important if you are trying to learn about available treatments or to connect with other women for mutual support and sharing. If you are researching medical or scientific information, always remember that nothing you read can substitute for conversations with your doctors. If you find something that interests you, make a note or print it out and talk with your doctor about it at your next visit. In general, it is better to seek out the sites of large and well-established organizations—for example, the Susan G. Komen Breast Cancer Foundation, the American Cancer Society, or the National Cancer Institute; the information on their sites will be accurate. Be wary of sites that seem to push too hard in one direction, that are critical of other approaches or resources, or that rely on commercial funding (although there are certainly some good health-information sites that are funded by for-profit businesses). Use your common sense and remember, as always, that something that sounds too good to be true probably is not true.

Participating in any kind of on-line support program or group can be challenging. I am especially wary of chat groups, which are open to anyone and not monitored by a professional, because they can contain all kinds of terrifying information. It is wonderful, of course, that there are ways for women to reach out to one another from around the world and to provide support and encouragement. Nonetheless, even though most participants in these groups are sharing from their hearts, their stories and words can be very upsetting or misleading. Remember as you read that you are seeing only what the writer is feeling and saying at this particular moment. You cannot be sure that her medical information is accurate or complete. It is very frightening to read of someone's recurrence or the progression of her disease when her situation appears to be much like your own. It is disturbing to read harsh criticism of medicine or doctors, because these charges, though based on one person's experiences, can make you uneasy about your own care. Even if there should be some validity to such judgments, you have no way to ascertain that, and a single individual's personal assessment is simply that: personal.

Much of the time women spend in chat rooms comes in the middle of the night. If you are upset and sleepless, turning on the computer and connecting with others may seem like a good idea; but always remember that no one's judgment is at its best at three in the morning and that *everything* seems worse at night. Reading letters from other women who are ill and scared will be even more traumatic than it would be in the daytime. If you cannot sleep, it is probably a better idea to make yourself a cup of herbal tea and read a light novel.

I do not mean to suggest that chat rooms, bulletin boards, and other on-line support networks are necessarily damaging; indeed, they can be especially valuable to women

who live in more-remote communities or who are otherwise isolated from others living with breast cancer. But I do
suggest that you begin your participation on-line with support groups that are monitored by a professional; check out
the Web sites of the major cancer organizations as a way to
find such groups. If these groups feel comfortable and safe
to you, you can then experiment with less-structured chat
rooms. And remember that you can always turn off the
computer and walk away if what you see disturbs you.

If you do participate in on-line chat rooms or bulletin
boards, I strongly recommend that you use a screen name
and that you are careful your e-mail address is not broad-
cast. Protect your privacy.

Stress-management programs can be of particular interest to women recovering from breast cancer. Many medical centers have programs in such departments as behavioral
medicine, family medicine, psychiatry, or social work.
These programs may be open to anyone who is interested in
learning better stress-management techniques, or they may
be designed to meet the needs of a particular population—
for example, people with hypertension, chronic pain, or
cancer. The goal of such programs is to teach cognitive and
behavioral strategies that enhance coping skills. Learning to
meditate, eliciting the relaxation response, or otherwise diminishing the body's natural reactions to stress may reduce
some physical symptoms associated with cancer and its
treatment, such as nausea or headaches. The programs last
for several weeks, and each session is usually devoted to a
single topic or strategy. The long-standing Mind–Body Cancer Program at my own medical center covers the relaxation

response, meditation, stretching, nutrition, yoga, biofeed-back, exercise, etc. Most people find participation in these programs very helpful. Even if some of the techniques may not seem useful or relevant, it is almost certain that everyone will find something of value among them.

Self-help groups differ from professionally facilitated groups. They are sometimes organized around a project or task and sometimes are intended to function as support groups. Both kinds are widely found and are often ex-tremely helpful. In some parts of the country, breast cancer self-help groups may be all that is available for women seek-ing a group experience, and they may be exactly what you need if you are looking for a way to connect with other women who are living with breast cancer. Still, there is one caveat to keep in mind. While there is never a guarantee that a professionally led group will be perfect, certain po-tential problems are more likely to arise when there is no professional group leader.

In general, groups can run into trouble if so much painful feeling is expressed that the participants are fright-ened and have no one to guide them toward resolution, or if the group rules are broken. In a breast cancer group, this can happen if a few members dominate the meetings and do not allow others time or space to speak. It can also arise when someone in the group has a worsening medical situa-tion and her fear and sadness terrify the other participants. Since a cardinal rule of group management is confidential-ity and mutual respect, it is also vital that "everything that is said in the room stays in the room." Without a group leader, it is sometimes hard to enforce this precept.

If you participate in a self-help or peer-led group, it

will be important to be especially alert to how it is affecting you. If you leave meetings feeling more upset than when you came, if you find that between meetings you are worrying about others in the group and have no way to alleviate these concerns, or if you feel disrespected or unheard in any way, this is not the right group for you. While these problems can also occur in a professionally led group, the odds are somewhat greater that they will not. The feelings associated with having breast cancer are so intense that they are both the best and the worst catalysts for producing a successful group. You will instantly feel connected to others living with the same fears, and you will instantly be vulnerable to their worries and to their situations.

In a professionally led support group, someone is there whose job it is to protect you and everyone else in the group. There is no way to guarantee that things won't be said that may be scary for you—this comes with the territory—but part of the leader's job is to make certain that everyone in the circle feels safe. In the groups that I facilitate, moments like this have arisen when someone in the group has a fear about a symptom, a recurrence, or a progression of her disease. At such times, it is always important to support the woman who is struggling, but it is just as important to attend to the needs of everyone there. We are careful to express our shared sorrow at someone's bad news, but we also express our own fear for ourselves. It is entirely appropriate and acceptable for someone to say, "My heart is breaking for you, but I am also so scared for me that I can barely breathe." Only by being able and even encouraged to share all aspects of our feelings can we honestly support one another *and* care for ourselves.

As you will have surmised, I am convinced that for many women (not all), a good group is the very best place to find support and understanding. When a group is working well, the members feel as Debbie does: "Sometimes I think how lonely it would be for me if I didn't have the love and support from our group. My whole life is so much better with all of you in it. I have learned so much from you." Or as Karen said: "I want to tell all of you that one thing I will be thankful for this year, and every day, has been the opportunity to know and be with you. I am hoping that for many years to come, I will be saying the same thing to all of you and that, as the years pass and we eat another thirty or so turkeys, we will look back on this time together with amazement and gratitude."

Working with these groups, and especially with the post-treatment breast cancer support groups, is one of the most rewarding parts of my job. Obviously the issues that these groups tackle are my issues, too. Although I am in the group as the leader and not as a participant, my heart is right in the midst of everyone else's. Their worries are my worries. Their grief is my grief. Their triumphs are my triumphs. I am blessed to be with them.

If you are looking for a professionally led support group, you can try asking your doctor or nurse for a referral. If they can't help you, call the largest hospital near you and ask to speak with an oncology social worker on their staff. She may be leading such a group; if she is not, she will certainly know of any that exist in the area. The American Cancer Society often maintains lists of support groups; call ACS's local number (listed in your telephone book's white pages) and ask for them. In the "Resources" section at the back of this book, you will find a list of national breast cancer organizations that may also maintain such lists. Other possibilities are the Association of Oncology Social Work (AOSW), the National Alliance of Breast Cancer Organizations (NABCO), the Wellness Community, the Susan G. Komen Breast Cancer Foundation Hotline, and Y-Me.

If you find a group and wonder whether it will be a good fit for you, there are some basic questions to ask. Is it a peer support group or is it professionally led? If it is professionally led, who is the leader and what are her qualifications? Who comes to the group? How old on average are the group members and where are they in their breast cancer continuum? Ideally, you want to find a group with other women who are similar to you in life stage as well as illness stage. If you have recently finished treatment and are trying to learn how to live your new life, you most certainly do not want to find yourself in a group that is comprised of women with metastatic disease. Finally, ask about any fee for the group. Most cancer support groups are offered as a community service and are free of charge. If there is a fee, it is possible that your insurance will cover the cost.

In remembering how uncertain she was about first attending a support group, Ginny, now a longtime member, said, "I am so happy that I went. No matter how I feel, this group of women makes me feel better, stronger, loved, and loving. No matter what the future brings, we will get through it together."

Nonetheless, groups are not right for everyone. If you

think that you would enjoy the fellowship of other women
but do not want the intensity of a support group, you might
consider joining a group or organization that is focused on
advocacy. Becoming politically active helps many women
feel more empowered and as though they are fighting back.
The National Breast Cancer Coalition and numerous state
Breast Cancer Coalitions are working toward increasing
funding and supporting research, public education, and
awareness of the need for early detection. The National
Coalition of Cancer Survivorship is a broader-based cancer
advocacy group that works with survivors' issues on a national and state or local level. The Susan G. Komen Breast
Cancer Foundation is the largest private funding source of
breast cancer research and community-based programs.
The Komen Foundation sponsors the Race for the Cure in
many cities and is always looking for volunteers to help
with this event and other fund-raising activities. There may
also be local organizations in your area that are raising
money, supporting educational efforts, or directly assisting
women with breast cancer and their families. All of them
could use your help.

You may also decide that it would be helpful to work
with a psychotherapist. Chapter 3 discussed post-traumatic
stress disorder (PTSD) and its connection to the trauma of
breast cancer. It also noted that many women struggle with
some degree of depression and distress after cancer and
would be helped by working with a therapist who is knowledgeable about breast cancer, its treatment, and the normal
process of psychological recovery. If, several months after
completing treatment, you find that you are having diffi-

culty sleeping, are often tearful and anxious, or are thinking much of the time about the possibility of recurrence and death, you should consider seeing a therapist. All of these feelings are normal in your circumstances, but you don't have to struggle through them alone. Again, you can ask your doctor or nurse for a referral to a therapist who is experienced with psycho-oncology.

There are many competent psychotherapists, but some of them know little or nothing about the issues surrounding breast cancer. It is probably not in your best interest right now to work with such individuals. The intensity of your feelings, your fear, and your grief may be misinterpreted by a therapist who has not had experience with other breast cancer survivors. She might not realize, for example, that your physical fatigue is a normal part of recovery and interpret it instead as a sign of depression. You should not be spending your precious therapy time and dollars educating your therapist about breast cancer.

All teaching hospitals and cancer centers, as well as many community hospitals, employ oncology social workers. Often, you do not have to be a medical patient at the facility to become a psychotherapy client of the oncology social worker. Call and ask. If she cannot see you at the hospital, ask if she has a private practice. You may also find it useful to ask other women who have had breast cancer about their experiences with therapy and therapists. Someone you sat next to in the radiation-therapy waiting room may know an experienced therapist to suggest. The most important thing is not to settle for second best or for someone whom you do not instinctively trust and like. The personal chemistry is very important. The hard work of psychother-apy takes place within the context of a human connection; it needs to be the right match for you. Like all other im-portant human relationships, you will know if it is right. Trust your instincts.

18

Spirituality and Faith

For each of us, our beliefs, our faith, and our prayers are wholly personal. Some do not identify with any formal spiritual tradition, finding other ways to seek meaning in life; for others, ritual and belief give strength and sustenance. But a diagnosis of cancer brings fear, and fear brings the need for hope—and it is my perception that faith seems inexorably bound up with hope; each begets the other. When we discover that we have breast cancer, we are not only afraid and sad, we are also filled with tremulous hope that is easily shaken and sometimes less easily strengthened. Moving through the months of treatment, we cradle that hope in our hearts and we cling to any words, any omens, and any feelings that can sustain it. We hope for an easy time with the treatment; we hope that the hard days will pass quickly; most of all, we hope that we will be lucky and go on to live long and well. Faith reassures us that all of this is possible and asks only that we believe. Belief does not require certainty; you only have to imagine it could be.

I have come to believe that faith lives where the heart is at home. Cancer pushes us hard to find our spiritual home. Throughout time and throughout the world, people have found sacred ground. In many cultures, it is where one's ancestors have walked the earth and are now buried. In others, it is places of special beauty where it is easy to imagine that spirits reside. Where there are both dawn and sunset, where we can love the night as well as the sunlight, where our minds are at peace and our souls at rest, there is sacred ground. We understand that this ground may literally be a place we plant our feet or simply a way of guiding our hearts and comforting our minds. Whatever it is, finding and consecrating it is a lifelong process and requires appreciation of where we have been, where we are standing, and—perhaps most importantly—where we are going. The journey's end may never be in sight as we travel unmapped paths.

There are many ways to find meaning in life and beliefs that sustain us. Each of us discovers what it is that holds and nurtures our own hearts and souls, and each of us will embark on our own journey. For me, that journey began in those first terrible days, when I found myself drawn to church and to nature. I had not attended church services with any regularity for many years; I still don't. But that first week, I went several times into an empty chapel. There I knelt and asked for grace and for courage. I did not dare to presume to ask for cure. Asking for help in managing whatever lay before me seemed the most that I could manage. February in Massachusetts is cold and dark and usually snowy. I recall once lying on the frozen ground in my back-yard, digging my nails into the snow and wishing that I could reach through to the earth itself. Pressed against the ground, I asked for grace and I asked for courage. It occurred to me then and it occurs to me now that lying on the ground may have been an unconscious symbolic act. Certainly I was fearful that in the near future I would be lying beneath that ground. Was I trying to master that terror? Was I practicing? Was I suggesting to the gods that above was better than below?

One of my older brothers is an Episcopal minister. He lives hundreds of miles away and is infrequently in Boston, but the week of my surgery he happened to be here for a conference. When my husband and I arrived at the hospital in the predawn dark, he was waiting for us. I had not expected to see him. He hugged me, and then he wrapped both of his hands around mine, looked deeply into my eyes, and asked God to be with me. That prayer and his faith comforted and kept me.

I believe in the power and importance of rituals. Therefore, my husband and I planned to mark the fifth anniversary of my diagnosis on Mount Desert Island, the place we love best. Before dawn we rose and bundled up against the Maine cold. We had hoped to greet this morning from the summit of Cadillac Mountain; not having been there before in midwinter, we were unaware the road was closed and the climb too long and icy in the predawn. Discovering this, we scouted another spot—easier to reach—from which we would meet the morning. We had not planned together what would happen once we scrambled over snow and rocks to the shore of the ocean. We had not talked about what we might say or do as the first light turned the sea to silver and the reborn sky burst open with gold.

It turned out that I brought music. He brought readings. Together we brought five years of grace, of intermittent terror, of deep sadness and deeper joy, and together we found strength that filled our hearts.

It is now three and a half years past that winter dawn. As I write this, I sit not far from that spot, in the summer sun, and gaze again at the sea and the mountains. We return each summer to this place; this island in Maine has become my sanctuary. Hiking here is prayer. When walking its wooded trails, I gaze heavenward and see a cathedral in the treetops. When I look down at the twisted and intertwined roots, I see the past and the triumph of life in the sprigs of green pushing through tiny crevices in the rock. When I spot a lone red fox on the hill or a single iris abloom on a boulder, I recognize miracles.

For many of us, it would be difficult, if not impossible, to have a potentially life-threatening illness and not think about God. What most marks us after cancer is the absolute recognition of our mortality, the end of any possible denial of our own death. We think not only about where we have been but also about where we are going. The central questions that have engaged men and women for all time are now ours. As one of my patients said to me recently, "I hope and usually believe that I am going to be okay. Sometimes I do get scared, and then I remember what I have already been through. My faith sustains me. I would never have thought that I could manage surgery and chemotherapy and radiation and feeling so ill, and I did. If the future brings me more cancer, I now know that somehow I will manage."

I have known many women who returned to the worship of their childhood after a cancer diagnosis. The familiar rituals bring comfort. Ann, a thirty-five-year-old mother of two young children, had been raised a Catholic but had married a non-Catholic man and not been to church for many years. As she struggled both to physically manage the travails of her treatment and to find meaning in her emotional pain, she was inexorably drawn to church. At first she entered the building at times when she knew she would be alone. Then she attended crowded services but always sat alone in the back, avoiding conversation with others. On one especially difficult day, she entered the church and sat silently in a pew, tears on her cheeks and eyes closed. She was startled by a touch on her hand and opened her eyes to see a very old woman standing close to her. "Welcome home," said the woman, who then turned and walked away.

Emily told me of riding in the hospital elevator after her final radiation treatment. She was bald, exhausted by months of treatment, and very frightened about her future. Her only companion in the elevator was a tiny, hunched-over elderly woman who stared straight ahead. As she was about to get off before Emily, she turned to look into her eyes, raised her fist in the air, and shook it for emphasis: "Never, ever, ever give up," she said.

Kayla, a sixty-five-year-old dancer whose daughter had been killed in an automobile accident many years earlier, went to a waterfall on the river near her home whenever her spirits were their lowest. Without fail, she told me, no matter what time of year it was, if she sat very still on a particular boulder, a butterfly would land on her shoulder.

Donna, walking from her car to her front door late in

the evening before her mastectomy, paused for a moment and asked for a sign. Looking up, she saw a shooting star blaze across the heavens.

If we are at all open, signs and meanings will find us.

It can be especially difficult to be open when we are angry and frightened. Some women believe that their cancer must be a punishment for sins in their lives. They wonder if they are being punished for an abortion or an extramarital affair or being unkind to aged parents or neglectful of the religion in which they were raised. Since my own childhood religion did not include a belief in divine retribution related directly to sin, I am able to see such fears as one more way of trying to understand and make sense of the uncontrollable.

While it does not accord with my own understanding of God, I am respectful of those who feel differently. If you find that you are struggling with this issue, I strongly urge you to find a priest or rabbi or minister with whom you can speak. If you worry that your own clergyperson may not be reassuring in this regard, you might consider searching for someone else. Choosing to speak with someone different does not mean that you are abandoning your own religion or your congregation. It means only that you are working hard toward finding redemption and peace and that you may need different experiences and different views to help you get there.

Another common belief is that "God gives us only what we can bear." Again, I understand that this view may be reassuring to those who believe that God knows our capabilities, and if He thinks I can do this, then surely I can find a way to do so.

It was very helpful to me some years ago to know and work with Elizabeth, a thirty-five-year-old minister who had breast cancer. She listened carefully one evening at a support group as another woman spoke at length of the many sorrows her family had had to endure and her own aggressive breast cancer now. When she ended saying that "God gives us only what we can carry," Elizabeth virtually lunged out of her chair. "That is such *crap!*" she exclaimed. "God gives some of us far more than we can carry. He makes mistakes." Coming from an ordained woman of God, these were powerful words indeed. I could see the lightness begin in the others' eyes. Perhaps it was acceptable to feel that the burden was too heavy. Maybe it was acceptable to be angry with God and to question His judgment. To hear from Elizabeth that God, too, makes mistakes was deeply relieving.

A cancer diagnosis is the beginning of many life changes. We are forced to recognize the omnipresent nature of endings and of loss. We lose any gauze shield of denial or special protection that we might have imagined existed around us. We begin to look at the world in different ways and are likely to truly behold it for the first time. All the clichés about smelling the roses become real. We truly see the dew on the blossoms and the colors of the sunset. And, even if we have never done so before, we start to think about our mortality.

Many of us believe that faith and spirituality do not have to be bound up in formal religion. Others firmly believe the converse: that a formal commitment to and affiliation with a particular religion is necessary and that community found as part of a congregation is invaluable. If you feel a longing for a church home, this is certainly a good time to start looking. All synagogues, churches, and mosques welcome visitors, and you can attend services wherever you wish. You may find that the devotions of your childhood feel most comfortable or you may find that, as an adult, you feel more at home in an entirely different place. The search for the right church or temple is not so different from the search for the right doctors or hospital. Talk to your friends. Ask questions. Read. Speak directly with the priest or the rabbi. And listen to your heart and to the moment it tells you that you are at home.

You will find that all of us, regardless of our particular beliefs, share much in common. Karen, an observant Jewish woman, found her spiritual home in a Catholic shrine. Telling me about this rather surprising choice, she said, "Mary was a Jewish mother just like me. I talk to her the way I talk to my friends."

If you undertake a spiritual journey, you may also find your way home along other paths. It is enormously reassuring to find that others have shared your thoughts and beliefs. This can help you feel less alone and more a part of a long tradition. Learning about Eastern religions, Islam, the ancient beliefs of Africans or Native Americans or other peoples may bring you much comfort.

My own core belief is that all of us are searching for truth and believing in the same God. There are, they say, no atheists in foxholes. There are few women with cancer who are not, at the very least, looking for faith and hope. Finding our sacred ground, our soulful home, the words that become our prayer, is a lifelong process. We might even consider ourselves fortunate to have begun at this time. If we stay well and go on to live long and healthy lives, we most certainly will enrich our days by what we have been taught by our time with cancer. Being forced to look straight at the tiger and not flinch gives us the chance to see the flicker of God in the tiger's eyes. What each of us sees, recognizes, and names is unique. What we share with one another and with all living creatures is universal and timeless.

19

Life After Breast Cancer

Shortly after my diagnosis, a friend sent me a card that read: *When you have come to the end of all you have ever known and around you is only darkness, faith is knowing one of two things will happen. Either you will find ground under your feet or you will grow wings to fly.* These words became so important to me that I later incorporated them into my wedding vows. Being diagnosed with a potentially life-threatening illness means the end of everything we have ever known. The world looks very different, and our place in it feels much less secure. Slowly we find our feet, stand erect, and start down the twisting path that lies ahead. Darkness lurks behind the curves and the destination is uncertain. Faith happens. It must. And each of us, in our own way, stumbling at first, finds that we have ground under our feet or wings to fly.

This is a time of thanksgiving, of harvesting what we have sown. The lives that we live after cancer are born of all that has come before. Forged by the pain of our experience, we are stronger. We have learned about ourselves and been tested in ways that we never dreamed. We have cherished our families and our friends, trusted our doctors, and reached out to help one another. We have examined our lives and our choices and begun to establish ourselves as we wish to be. It is impossible and inappropriate to tell a newly diagnosed woman, who is in the throes of the initial crisis, that good is likely to come of her breast cancer. But remember the psychiatrist who liked to say, "Adults only grow on the rack." We have been stretched and we have grown. The fact that this is the truth is a strong statement about human resilience.

Is it worth it? Absolutely not! But the experiences of being diagnosed with cancer, living through very difficult physical treatments, and somehow learning to manage and accept the psychological challenges give us a chance to live more fully. The phrase *living out loud* is sometimes used to describe the intensity and passion of life after cancer. There is no time or patience left for living in silence.

Perhaps the loveliest story about these feelings is one that I heard from one of my well-traveled patients. Several years after the completion of her breast cancer treatment, she went to Peru with her family. A highlight of their trip was a visit to the temples at Machu Picchu, the ancient Inca site in Peru. It was a warm day and they climbed the steep temple steps with a group of American and Peruvian hikers. The Americans, she said, scrambled ahead and moved quickly and steadily toward the summit. The Peruvians lagged behind and periodically sat down to rest. One of the American men called down to them, saying, "What are you doing? We're trying to get a move on here." The response was, "We are waiting. We need to give our souls time to catch up."

That image has stayed with me and beautifully frames the concept of our new lives. Physically, we have been forced to keep pace with the treatments and with our bodies. Behaviorally, we have tended to our family and work responsibilities and tried to carry on normally. Our lives have been changed in many ways and we have tried to be understanding and flexible about our possibilities. Our hearts, our souls, however, need time to catch up. Their rhythm is far less steady and certain than the rate of hair growth or the return of energy.

Let me share the thoughts of a number of women I have known.

From Laurie: "I realized what a good life I have. No more taking myself, my life partner, my friends, my health, my accomplishments, all the daily gifts from unexpected places for granted. I learned that 'alone' is a lie. Living through cancer gives me automatic membership in a community of others who accept, see, hear, and understand each other in a basic way that isn't possible without belonging to this club. My loneliness and sense of wanting to but not really belonging to any group has eased up in a major way. At first I thought that everyone with cancer was conferred with sainthood. I was and am so proud of how we all tried to fight our way back to life and how many of us succeeded. By now I have noticed that I am still capable of acting like a jerk and so are the others, yet I am wired to like anyone else who is living with cancer."

From Perry: "I've had breast cancer twice, with seven

years between the two, and now seven years since the second diagnosis. The first time I didn't make changes in my life. The second diagnosis was a dramatic wake-up call: I might not live as long as I'd hoped, so we'd better make the most of my time. I was fifty-three when I was diagnosed the second time and had been married for a year to a man whose first wife had died of cancer! After treatment and some time to recover, my husband and I decided that I would quit my job as a newspaper editor. I needed more free time, time to reach out to others with cancer, time to write a book about hope and cancer. We also sold our house in the suburbs, bought a house at the beach, and rented an apartment in the city. Ever since, we've played as much as we can, within reason. We try not to spend time doing anything that does not please us or produce positive results. This post-cancer time has been the best time of my life. I'm focused, very alive, and am challenged by the work that I do."

From Karen: "I sat down this week to my art, the first time I have tried to do my work since my diagnosis. I realized that I am sitting in the same spot, but that I am transfigured."

From Marilyn: "Oddly, I don't worry about the future. I believe I have received the best possible treatment and am truly grateful. I know there are no guarantees; this cancer will either come back or it won't. It's as simple as that. So I don't worry about the things that I can't control. Except for the doctors' appointments on my calendar and the mysteriously missing right breast, I am hard pressed to remember that I had cancer."

From Betty: "What a difference a year makes! Last year

my bed was made and my laundry was always caught up, but I had no garden. This year, my laundry is all over the basement floor, but my garden is in full bloom."

From Ann: "Much of my dissatisfaction comes from not meeting what I perceive as other peoples' expectations that I be fine, over the cancer, back to my old self. That old self does not exist anymore; I have changed profoundly. What counts is how I think of and deal with my own life. I can be peaceful and proud of doing the best I can, focusing on all that is good, if I choose to do so."

From Julia: "I think my life is somehow supposed to get normal again, but I certainly don't know exactly how or when that is going to happen!"

In fact, it happens slowly, in fits and starts, with lots of backsliding. You are living through the end of who you were and the life you had, and the beginning of something else. You are learning both who you are and what your life will become. My experience has been that most women do not make major changes in the structure of their lives, although there are exceptions. I did know a dentist who sold her practice and bought a larger sailboat. She and her partner sailed off to the Caribbean with their eyes on more-distant horizons. I have also known a number of women who changed their jobs, started to paint or write or garden, made a commitment to a love relationship or left a relationship that wasn't working. Most of us, however, make small external changes; it is the internal ones that are profound. We focus more on the way we look at the world and our place in it and much less on what others think. That way is related most of all to our intense commitment to ourselves and to those we love; rarely does it relate to material success and things.

Terri, a lovely young woman who had just completed her chemotherapy, reminded me that the whole concept of eventually feeling normal seems impossible at the start. Like all of us in those first days, she was struggling with her physical health and trying to look toward the future, but the treatment experience was far too recent and raw for her to imagine that life could feel different and better. If you, too, are at that stage, let me repeat that the passage of time will bring you to a very different psychological place. Just because you are not now able to imagine feeling sturdy and normal, that day will come.

It will be a different you, however. In the beginning, you probably were impatient to "get your life back" and did not realize that your previous life was lost to you forever. Although you can experience even more-intense joy and delight than ever before, you will never again be carefree. There is a bittersweet quality to all important markers and events. I remember being asked during a support-group meeting, "What are we supposed to celebrate now?" The only answer is "Everything." How you celebrate is up to you, but celebrate you must.

For a couple of years leading up to my fiftieth birthday, I was too superstitious to let myself think about how to mark this half-century anniversary. Thinking or talking about it made me very anxious. Finally, several months before the day, my husband said, "Unless you are hit by a truck, you are going to be alive on your fiftieth birthday, and we are going to celebrate." At first reluctantly, and then with growing enthusiasm, we planned a small dinner for family and close friends at a lovely hotel in Boston. This, after all, was an important birthday that six years earlier I had not let myself believe I would have. This wonderful evening felt very special to me and, I hope, to my guests. The best part was my decision to write letters to each person who was coming and use them as place cards at the tables. For days before the event, I thought about what each person meant to me, how grateful I was for that unique relationship, and what I wanted to say in appreciation and love. Writing these letters was a wonderful opportunity to give thanks to my family and friends and to make certain that there would never be things left unsaid to those people who mean the most to me. You may remember my earlier story about the rings, now our wedding bands, that my husband and I had made immediately following my diagnosis. For this important birthday, he returned to the same goldsmith and asked that a necklace be made in the same design. It symbolizes for us both the unending circle of our love and our lives and the thanksgiving we share for these years together.

My life is far different than it would have been if I had not had breast cancer. I am physically changed, but I am emotionally transformed. The grand goal of never again becoming irritated by small things is, of course, often not met. I tell my new patients that one way they will recognize the return of better mental health and normalcy is when they again find themselves angry in traffic or frustrated with a husband's habit of throwing his dirty clothes on the floor. We are not saints; we are intensely and gratefully human. But we have learned to be gentle with ourselves and with those we love. How we cherish our husbands, our partners, our children, our friends! We do sometimes stop to smell a rose or pull off the road to watch the sun set into the ocean. If we walk in the forest early in the autumn, we are aware of the crunch and the sweet smell of the leaves beneath our feet. If we walk the same path later, we notice that they have turned brown and the sweet smell has gone. The death of the year surrounds us, but we have faith in the spring. The small animals have disappeared; we know some will never return, but most will reappear in the spring green and some will be accompanied by new life. We find a solace and promise in the natural rhythms that surround and carry us.

When I give talks, I sometimes conclude with suggestions for life that I have learned from so many cancer patients I have known. The list includes:

** In your garden, plant perennials.
** Keep current. Pay attention to your relationships.
** Find something frivolous that makes you happy and do it often. For me, this has meant keeping fresh flowers in my house and getting a weekly manicure—things I had never once done before my diagnosis.
** Live a little beyond your budget.
** Love as much as you can and then learn to love even more.

There is one very serious suggestion that is the essence of how we hope to live. Although most of the people with whom I have worked have done well, I have sadly known and loved and lost too many to cancer. Watching them, being with them through the progression of their illness, I have learned what really matters. We have to think about how we want to live and we have to consider how we will someday want to die. All of us must learn how to live so we will know how to die. Equally important, in learning how to die, we will know how to live.

As I write this, it is almost ten years since my cancer was diagnosed in February 1993. I am still sometimes afraid and sometimes sad, though far from always and certainly less often than in the past. Because I spend my days working in an oncology unit and am married to an oncologist, cancer surrounds me, and I am extremely respectful of its hated power and guile. My life's work has become my life, and, through these last years, this life has become familiar and normal. I have become comfortable in my changed skin. For a long time now, I have brushed a full head of hair and gone running most mornings. The golden retriever puppy that we brought home six days after my final chemotherapy treatment is now a ninety-pound graying-at-the-muzzle member of the family. I remember looking at him on my young daughter's lap and wondering which of us would survive the other. I remember hoping that he would be a comfort to her if I died. Blessedly, he has been a comfort to us both, and he has not been called upon to provide solace to that kind of broken heart.

The search for meaning remains central to my life. I continuously reflect on what has happened to me as I try to move forward. My longtime philosophical model of Sisyphus, of recognizing and accepting how and why I continue to push the boulder up the hill, has been joined with the story from Genesis of Jacob wrestling with the angel of God and finally emerging scathed, triumphant, and blessed.

I am proud to be part of a very special sisterhood, and grateful for my companions on the journey.

In writing this book, I have tried to say to you on paper what I would say to you in person. I would like to be able to look into your eyes and feel the connection between us. I wish that you could take a rock from my basket, keep it close, and someday add another rock to the collection that will become another woman's talisman. I wish that I could have the personal opportunity to promise you that time helps, that you will feel better, and that shining life beckons at the end of your tunnel. It would bring me much joy later to watch you reach back your hand toward the darkness to support someone else as she begins the journey. Woman to woman, heart to heart, we pass it on.

We close our support groups with this prayer written by Jan Montgomery, an extraordinary woman who is living with metastatic breast cancer. It is a fitting way to close this book, too.

We are thankful to be with each other today, knowing that both our pain and our good news are truly shared by others. We ask that where there is heartache we will be given understanding and love. We especially hold all of our sisters in our hearts and wish them strength and comfort on difficult days. We pray for help to quiet our fears and raise our spirits. We ask for strength to forgive others as well as ourselves. We are thankful

for the care and support that we receive from each
other and we ask for both grace and grit to live
fully each and every day.

In the words of the traditional Jewish toast and blessing:

L'Chaim.
To Life.
In every way, choose life.

Afterword and Resources

Because the text contains many suggestions about organizations that might be helpful to you, this section is relatively short and simple. Information on the Internet changes constantly, and, as described in Chapter 17, your best approach is to explore well-known and established breast cancer sites.

Below are a number of reliable organizations that maintain very thorough and informative Web sites. You can start with any of them, use their links to other sites, and feel certain that you are reading accurate information.

The suggested books are an idiosyncratic collection of titles that I have especially liked; it is not intended to be an exhaustive bibliography of good books about breast cancer or other related subjects.

ORGANIZATIONS

These are all well-established and trustworthy organizations that have useful Web sites and may be directly contacted for other questions or information.

American Cancer Society
(ACS)
1599 Clifton Road, NE
Atlanta, Georgia 30329
800 ACS-2345
www.cancer.org

American Society of Clinical
Oncology (ASCO)
1900 Duke Street, Suite 200
Alexandria, Virginia 22314
703 299-0150
www.asco.org

Association of Oncology
Social Work (AOSW)
1211 Locust Street
Philadelphia, Pennsylvania
19107
215 545-8107
www.aosw.org

Cancer Care, Inc.
275 Seventh Avenue
New York, New York 10001
212 712-8080 or
800 813-4673
www.cancercare.org

Celebrating Life Organization
(for African-American
women)
PO Box 224076
Dallas, Texas 75222
800 207-0992
www.celebratinglife.org

Fertile Hope (helping cancer
patients with fertility)
PO Box 624
New York, New York 10014
888 994-HOPE
www.fertilehope.org

Living Beyond Breast Cancer
10 East Athens Avenue,
Suite 204
Ardmore, Pennsylvania 19003
610 645-4567
www.lbbc.org

Mary-Helen Mautner Project
for Lesbians with Cancer
1707 L Street NW, Suite 230
Washington, D.C. 20036
202 332-5536
www.mautnerproject.org

National Alliance of Breast
Cancer Organizations
(NABCO)
9 East 37th Street, 10th floor
New York, New York 10016
212 889-0606 or
888 80-NABCO
www.nabco.org
Note: NABCO publishes an
excellent annual breast-cancer
resource book that is available
directly from them.

National Breast Cancer
Coalition (NBCC)
1707 L Street NW,
Suite 1060
Washington, D.C. 20036
202 296-7477 or
800 622-2838
www.stopbreastcancer.org

National Cancer Institute
(NCI)
31 Center Drive
Bethesda, Maryland 20892
301 435-3848 or
800 422-6237
www.nci.nih.gov
Note: NCI is a constituent of
the National Institutes of
Health; its informational
Web site, *http://
cancernet.nci.nih.gov,* is superb.

National Center for
Complementary and
Alternative Medicine
PO Box 8218
Silver Spring, Maryland 20907
800 644-6226
www.nccam.nih.gov

National Lymphedema Network
1611 Telegraph Avenue,
Suite 1111
Oakland, California 94612
800 541-3259
www.lymphnet.org

OncoLink
University of Pennsylvania
Cancer Center
www.oncolink.com

Quackwatch: Your Guide to
Health Fraud, Quackery, and
Intelligent Decisions
http://www.quackwatch.com
Note especially "A Special
Message for Cancer Patients
Seeking 'Alternative'
Treatments."

The Susan G. Komen Breast
Cancer Foundation
5005 LBJ Freeway, Suite 250
Dallas, Texas 75244
972 855-1600 or
1-800-I'M AWARE (helpline)
www.komen.org

SusanLoveMD.Com
PO Box 846
Pacific Palisades, California
90272
310 230-1712
www.susanlovemd.com

Y-Me National Breast Cancer
Organization
212 West Van Buren Street,
Suite 500
Chicago, Illinois 60607
312 986-8338
www.y-me.org
Y-Me maintains a twenty-four-
hour toll-free hotline. Call
them anytime at
800 221-2141.

Young Survival Coalition
(survivors under 40)
PO Box 528
52A Carmine Street
New York, New York 10014
212 206-6610
www.youngsurvival.org
This organization, with both
national and local chapters, is
especially important and
valuable for young women
with breast cancer.

BOOKS

Special and thoughtful books about cancer, illness, or life

Albom, Mitch. *Tuesdays with Morrie.* New York: Doubleday, 1997.
If you have somehow missed this book, you need to read it now.

Broyard, Anatole. *Intoxicated by My Illness.* Foreword by Oliver
Sacks. New York: Clarkson Potter, 1992. A wonderful and intelligent book about illness and patient/doctor relationships.

Frank, Arthur. *At the Will of the Body.* Boston: Houghton Mifflin, 1991. A profound and moving book of life and illness.

Lynn, Joanne, M.D. *Handbook for Mortals: Guidance for People
Facing Serious Illness.* London: Oxford University Press, 1999. A
book that is rich in material, including poetry and photographs.

Nessim, Susan, and Judith Ellis. *Can Survive: Reclaiming Your Life After Cancer.* Boston: Houghton Mifflin, 2000. An excellent resource guide for survivors of all types of cancer.

Oliver, Mary. *New and Selected Poems.* Boston: Beacon Press, 1992. Poetry as metaphor for life's meaning.

Sontag, Susan. *Illness As Metaphor.* New York: Anchor Books, 1990. The classic book that strips cancer of its stigma.

Selected titles about breast cancer

Lorde, Audre. *The Cancer Journals.* San Francisco: Aunt Lute Books, 1980. Reflections on her breast cancer by this self-described "black lesbian poet warrior."

Love, Susan, M.D., with Karen Lindsey. *Dr. Susan Love's Breast Book.* Third Edition. Cambridge, Mass.: Perseus Publishing, 2000. The classic reference book.

MacPherson, Myra. *She Came to Live Out Loud.* New York: Scribner, 1999. A moving and thoughtful book about a young woman dying of breast cancer and her family.

Porter, Margit Esser. *Hope Lives!* Peterborough, New Hampshire: h.i.c. publishing, 2000. A lovely small book of quotes from many women surviving breast cancer.

Sigler, Hollis. *Hollis Sigler's Breast Cancer Journal.* New York: Hudson Hills Press, 1999. In addition to the text, this book is a gorgeous collection of sixty of the author's paintings about her breast cancer experience.

Springer, Melissa. *A Tribe of Warrior Women: Breast Cancer Survivors.* Birmingham, Alabama: Crane Hill Publishers, 1996. A unique and beautiful photographic book.

Stabiner, Karen. *To Dance with the Devil: The New War on Breast Cancer: Politics, Power, People.* New York: Delacorte Press, 1997. The politics of breast cancer.

Weiss, Marisa C., M.D., and Ellen Weiss. *Living Beyond Breast Cancer: A Survivor's Guide for When Treatment Ends and the Rest of Your Life Begins.* New York: Times Books, 1998. An encyclopedic book about life after breast cancer treatment.

Complementary therapies

American Cancer Society. *American Cancer Society's Guide to Complementary and Alternative Cancer Methods.* Atlanta, Georgia: American Cancer Society, 2000. An encyclopedic guide to traditional and complementary therapies.

Gordon, James S., M.D., and Sharon Curtin. *Comprehensive Cancer Care: Integrating Alternative, Complementary, and Conventional Therapies.* Cambridge, Massachusetts: Perseus Publishing, 2001. Another thorough guide to evaluating and choosing treatments and practitioners.

Lerner, Michael. *Choices in Healing.* Cambridge, Massachusetts: The MIT Press, 1996. A thorough and thoughtful resource that is widely appreciated by both conventional and alternative-medicine practitioners.

O'Toole, Carole, with Carolyn B. Hendricks, M.D. *Healing Outside the Margins: The Survivor's Guide to Integrative Cancer Care.* Washington, D.C.: Lifeline Press, 2002. Written by a survivor of inflammatory breast cancer, this book presents a step-by-step plan for evaluating complementary-care therapies and making careful choices.

Physical recovery

Davis, Sherry Lebed. *Thriving After Breast Cancer: Essential Healing Exercises for Body and Mind.* New York: Broadway Books, 2002. An original and most helpful collection of stretches and dance-like movements to restore physical flexibility and well-being.

Toglia, Annie. *Staying Abreast: Rehabilitation Exercises for Breast Cancer Surgery.* This book is available at *www.stayingabreast.com.* Comprehensive information and exercises for regaining strength, flexibility, and comfort after breast surgery.

Family and marital concerns

Donner, C. B. *Confronting the Cow: A Young Family's Struggle with Breast Cancer, Loss, and Rebuilding.* Durham, North Carolina: Moonlight Publishing, 2000. A moving account of a family's experience with the illness and eventual death of their wife/mother at age 36.

Fincannon, Joy L., R.N., M.S., and Katherine V. Bruss, Psy.D. *Couples Confronting Cancer: Keeping Your Relationship Strong.* Atlanta, Georgia: American Cancer Society, 2002. Like other titles published by the American Cancer Society, this book of advice for couples dealing with cancer is wide-ranging and practical.

Harpham, Wendy S., M.D. *When a Parent Has Cancer: A Guide to Caring for Your Children.* New York: HarperCollins, 1997. Includes a separate illustrated book for children.

Heiney, Sue P., Ph.D., R.N., Joan F. Hermann, M.S.W., L.S.W., Katherine V. Bruss, Psy.D., and Joy L. Fincannon, R.N., M.S. *Cancer in the Family.* Atlanta, Georgia: American Cancer Society, 2001. A very useful guide for families, written by oncology clinicians.

Sexuality

Altman, C. *You Can Be Your Own Sex Therapist.* New York: Casper Publishing, 1997. An excellent book for individuals and couples experiencing sexual difficulties.

Goodwin, A. J., and M. E. Agronin. *A Woman's Guide to Overcoming Sexual Fear and Pain.* Oakland, California: New Harbinger

Publications, 1997. A very helpful guide that includes written exercises, directions for sensate exercises, specific sexual directions and suggestions.

Kahane, Deborah Hobler. *No Less a Woman: Femininity, Sexuality, and Breast Cancer.* Alameda, California: Hunter House, Inc., 1995. The author is a breast cancer survivor.

Rako, S. *The Hormone of Desire: The Truth About Testosterone, Sexuality, and Menopause.* New York: Three Rivers Press, 1996. A concise and informative book.

Schover, Leslie R., Ph.D. *Sexuality and Fertility After Cancer.* New York: John Wiley and Sons, Inc., 1997. The classic in the field.

Insurance, legal, and financial issues

Hoffman, Barbara, J.D., editor. *A Cancer Survivor's Almanac: Charting Your Journey,* Third Edition. New York: John Wiley and Sons, 2003. This is an excellent reference volume from the National Coalition for Cancer Survivorship (*www.canceradvocacy.org*).

Landay, David S., J.D. *Be Prepared: The Complete Financial, Legal, and Practical Guide for Living with a Life-Challenging Condition.* New York: St. Martin's Press, 1998. Superb and essential.

Index

Abandonment, sense of, 31

Acupuncture, 121, 125, 127–128

Acute crisis, 21–22

Adaptation, 22–23

Adjuvant chemotherapy, 24–25, 170

Adoption, 168–169

Adriamycin, 68

Advocacy, 260

Ahles, Tim A., 77–78

Alternative treatments, 121

Alzheimer's disease, 78–79

American Association of Sex Educators, Counselors, and Therapists, 162

American Cancer Society (ACS), 232, 253, 258–259

American Society of Clinical Oncologists (ASCO), 87

American Society of Clinical Oncology (ASCO), 87–88, 230–231

Americans with Disabilities Act of 1990 (ADA), 217–218

Anger, 13, 20, 45, 47, 48, 133, 249

Antidepressants, 158

Anxiety, 14, 20, 31, 46, 70, 90, 127, 133, 222–223, 227, 249

Appetite, loss of, 21

Arimidex, 113

Aromatase inhibitors, 103–104, 112–114, 170

Ashkenazi Jews, 221, 223, 225
Aspirin, 109–110
Association of Oncology
    Social Work (AOSW), 259
Axillary surgery, 55–56, 64

Balance, search for, 33–35
Beth Israel Deaconess Medical
    Center, 8, 64
Biopsy, endometrial, 109
Blood chemistries, 94
Blood clots, 109–110
Blood tests:
    for CA-125 protein, 228
    fertility and, 171
    for genetic testing, 223–224
    medical follow-up and, 89,
        90, 93–96
Bone pain, 87
Bone scans, 93
Books, 286–290
"Boosts," 56–57
BRCA1 gene, 220–221, 223,
    225, 226, 230, 231
BRCA2 gene, 221, 223, 225,
    226, 230, 231
Breast cancer genes:
    anxiety about genetic pre-
        disposition, 222–223
    prevalence of genetically
        based breast cancer,
        221–222
    testing for, 221, 223–234

blood test, 223–224
    decision making about,
        224–225, 232–234
    for-profit laboratory vs.
        medical center, 224
    implications of negative
        tests, 231–232
    implications of positive
        tests, 225–231
    information on, 232
Breast cancer hierarchy, 30
Breast Cancer Prevention
    Trial, 231
Breast cancer recurrence,
    86–89, 96–98, 246
    fear of, 96, 236–237, 244–
        248
    kinds of, 86–87, 239–244
Breast MRI, 92, 227
Breast reconstruction, 53–55
Breast self-examination, 87,
    96–97
Breast ultrasound, 91
Brewer's yeast, 64
Burnes, Michael J., 81

Cancer anniversary, marking,
    141–142
Cancer markers, 94–95
Cardiac complications, 68–69
CAT scans, 93
CBC (Complete Blood
    Count), 94

Center for the Study of Complementary Medicines, 120
Chemobrain, 77–80
Chemotherapy, 17–19, 28, 29, 52, 241
   adjuvant, 24–25, 170
   cardiac complications and, 68–69
   dental problems and, 81
   fertility and, 169–170
   hormonal therapies following, 116
   memory problems and, 77–80
   weight gain and, 58
Chest X rays, 92–93
Children, 175–190, 220–221, 250
Chinese herbs, 120
Chondroitin, 76
Clinical trials, 119, 238–239
Clothing, 53, 61, 64
Communication, 49
   about sex, 148–150
   about support, 250
   with friends, 204–205
   with husbands or partners, 132–135, 140, 148–150
Complementary therapies, 118–131
   acupuncture, 121, 125, 127–128
   vs. alternative treatments, 121
   data-based information on, 119–120
   evidence and, 119
   extent of use of, 121–122
   herbal medicine, 121, 126–127
   moments in continuum of care and interest in, 122–124
   nutrition and nutritional therapies, 128–130
   Reiki, 120–122, 128
   safety and, 120
   selecting practitioners, 124–125
   types of, 122
Counselors, 136–137
Cuticles, 66–67, 81
Cytoxan, 18

Dartmouth Medical School, 78
Decision making, 49
Dental problems, 80–81
Depression, 31, 46, 158, 249
Diagnosis of breast cancer, 12–14, 26, 122–123, 263
Diet, 65–66, 128–130
Dieting, 59–60
Disability insurance, 215–216
Discrimination, workplace, 216–219

Distant recurrence, 86–87
Divorce, 137–138

Earhart, Amelia, 246
Eastern medicine, 126–127
Eisenberg, David, 121
Emotions:
    fatigue and, 70
    finishing treatment and,
        15–16, 19–21, 28,
        30–32
    of husbands and partners,
        133, 135
    life after cancer and, 278
    normalcy of overpowering
        feelings, 47–48
    post-traumatic stress disor-
        der (PTSD) and, 45–46
    psychological-support
        services and, 44–45
    venting, 49
Endometrial biopsy, 109
Endometrial cancer, 107–109
Energy, low, 69–72
Equal Employment
    Opportunity Commission
    (EEOC), 218
Estriadol, 171
Estrogen, 59, 103, 106, 112–
    113, 127, 147, 155–159
Estrogen-receptor-negative
    breast cancer, 104, 105
Estrogen-receptor-positive

breast cancer, 104–106,
    155–156, 170, 226
Exercise, 61, 67, 72, 74
Eyebrows:
    loss of, 52
    makeup and, 37
    regrowth of, 63
Eyelashes:
    makeup and, 37
    regrowth of, 63
Eye shadow, 37

Faith, 251, 263–271
Family:
    aftermath of treatment
        and, 41–43
    children, 175–190, 220–
        221, 250
    husbands, See Husbands
    parents, 191–198, 250
Family and Medical Leave Act
    (FMLA), 218–219
Fatigue, 24, 69–72
Fear, 20, 45, 268
    of breast cancer recur-
        rence, 96, 236–237,
        244–248
    diagnosis of cancer and,
        13, 21, 25, 263
    of dying, 28, 43
Femara, 115
Fertility, 166–171
Flashbacks, 45

Follow-up, *See* Medical follow-up
Foreboding, sense of, 10–12
Friends:
  aftermath of treatment and, 41–43
  communicating with, 204–205
  losing, 199–200, 205
  medical follow-up and, 90–91
  reactions of, 199–203
  support from, 250
  in support groups, 204
FSH (follicle-stimulating hormone), 171

Ganz, Patricia, 76
Gass, Laurie Beth, 234–235
Genetic testing, 221
  blood test, 223–224
  decision making about, 224–225, 232–234
  for-profit laboratory vs. medical center, 224
  implications of negative tests, 231–232
  implications of positive tests, 225–231
  information on, 232
Glucosamine, 76
Goat's milk soap, 56

Grief, 13, 20, 21, 48
Gynecologists, 85, 162

Hair color, 62–64
Hair dye, 64
Hair growth, 31, 62–64
Hair loss, 52, 61–62
Headaches, 110
Health-care providers, attitudes of, 143–144
Health Insurance Portability and Accounting Act of 1996 (HIPAA), 213–214
Herbal medicine, 73–74, 121, 126
High-risk specialists, 225
Hope, 263
Hormonal therapies, 29, 58, 103–117
  aromatase inhibitors, 103–104, 112–114
  Tamoxifen, *See* Tamoxifen
Hormone-replacement therapy (HRT), 72, 73, 155–157
Hot flashes, 69, 72–75, 110, 115–116, 127, 156
Humor, sense of, 64
Husbands and partners, concerns of, 20, 43, 132–142, 250
  changes in the relationship, 139–142

Husbands and partners (*cont.*)
    communication and,
        132–135, 140
    counselors or therapists
        and, 136–137
    emotions and, 133, 135
    separation and divorce,
        137–138
    sexuality, *See* Sexuality
Hypnosis, 18
Hysterectomy, 109

Infection, signs of, 68
Infertility specialists, 168, 169
Intercourse:
    painful, 156–160
    position during, 160–161

"Jewish breast cancer gene," 221
Joint pain, 75–77
*Journal of the National Cancer
    Institute,* 226
Journals, 49, 189–190

Komen, Susan B., Breast
    Cancer Foundation, 253,
    259, 260

Leg cramps, 110
Lesbian couples, 142–145

LH (luteinizing hormone),
    171
Life after breast cancer,
    272–282
Life insurance, 215
"Living out loud," 273
Local recurrence, 86,
    239–241
Loprinzi, Charles, 73
Lorde, Audre, 245
Love, Susan, 222
Low energy, 69–72
Lubricants, vaginal, 159
Lumpectomy, 52, 64
Lupron, 170
Lymphatics, 64–65
Lymphedema, 64–68
Lymph nodes, 55, 64

Makeup tips, 36–37
Mammography, 87–88, 91,
    227
Manicures, 66–67
Mastectomy, 52, 53, 64, 151,
    226, 240
Masturbation, 155
Mayo Clinic, 226
Medical follow-up, 36,
    83–102
    American Society of Clini-
        cal Oncology (ASCO)
        guidelines for,
        87–88

blood tests, 89, 90, 93–96
bone scans, 93
breast cancer recurrence
    and, 86–89, 97–98
breast MRI, 92
breast self-examination,
    87, 96–97
breast ultrasound, 91
CAT scans, 93
changing doctors, 84–85
chest X rays, 92–93
doctor's domains and,
    85–86
mammography, 87–88, 91
MRI, 93
PET scan, 92
stress and, 90–91
summary, 101–102
Medical history, oral, 88
Medical insurance, 209–210,
    213–214
Memory problems, 77–80
Menopause, 58, 147, 155
Metastatic breast cancer,
    86–89, 240–244
Mind-Body Cancer Program,
    255–256
Montgomery, Jan, 281–282
Mood swings, 20–21, 45,
    110
Mortality, 236–238, 244–248
MRI, 93
    breast, 92, 227
Muscle stiffness, 75–77

"My Balancing Act" (Zorfass),
    33–35

Nail polish, 81–82
Nails, 66–67, 81–82
National Alliance of Breast
    Cancer Organizations
    (NABCO), 232, 259
National Breast Cancer Coali-
    tion (NBCC), 232, 260
National Cancer Institute
    (NCI), 120, 232, 253
National Coalition of Cancer
    Survivorship, 260
National Institutes of Health
    (NIH), 119, 155
Nausea, 18, 24, 90, 110, 125,
    127
Nervelike pains, 57
Nolvadex, See Tamoxifen
Nutrition and nutritional
    therapies, 128–130

Office "cancer magnet," 212
Oncologists, 86, 148, 162,
    244
Online chat rooms or support
    groups, 253–255
Oophorectomy, 226–227
Organizations, 284–286
Orgasm, 155, 158, 161
Osteoporosis, 114

Panic, 25
Parents, 191–198, 250
Partners, concerns of, *See*
  Husbands and partners,
  concerns of; Lesbian
  couples
Patient to Patient, Heart to
  Heart, 8
Peer-led groups, 256–257
Performance anxiety, 149
Pets, 50
PET scan, 92, 227
Physical effects of treatment,
  18–19, 24, 27
Physical examination, 88
Physical recovery, 51–82
  cardiac complications,
    68–69
  dental problems, 80–81
  fatigue and low energy,
    69–72
  hair growth, 62–64
  hair loss, 61–62
  hot flashes, 69, 72–75
  lymphedema, 64–68
  memory problems, 77–80
  muscle stiffness and joint
    pain, 75–77
  nails, 81–82
  post-radiation changes,
    56–58
  post-surgery changes,
    52–56
  timing of, 51–52

weight gain, 58–60
weight loss, 59–61
Physician-assisted suicide, 247
Polygenic women, 222
Post-radiation changes, 56–58
Post-surgery changes, 52–56
Post-traumatic stress disorder
  (PTSD), 45–46
Pregnancy, 166–174
Primary-care physician
  (PCP), 85, 86
Professional issues, 207–219
  disability insurance, 215–
    216
  disclosing your situation,
    209–210
  discrimination, 216–219
  evaluating priorities
    and perspectives
    concerning, 210–211
  expectations of colleagues,
    213
  life insurance, 215
  loss of self-confidence,
    208–209, 212
  medical insurance, 209–
    210, 213–214
  office "cancer magnet,"
    212
  timing of return to work,
    208
Professionally-led support
  groups, 257–259
Prostheses, 53

Psycho-educational or
    information groups,
    252–253
Psychological-support
    services, 44–45
Psychotherapy, 46–47,
    260–262
Pubic hair, 52, 63

Radiation recall, 57–58
Radiation therapy, 17–18, 28,
    29, 56–58
Reconstruction surgery, 53–
    55
Recurrent breast cancer, *See*
    Breast cancer recurrence
Redness, post-radiation,
    56–58
Reiki, 120–122, 128
Religion, 269–270
Replens, 159, 160
Retin-A, 160
Rituals, 16–17, 36, 265–
    267

Sadness, 13, 20, 28, 45, 70,
    158
Scalp massage, 64
Scars, 29, 151
Scar tissue, 57
Self-confidence, loss of, 208–
    209, 212

Self-help groups, 256–257
Self-image, 151
Sentinel-node biopsy
    procedure, 55
Separation, marital, 137–138
Sex therapists, 162
Sexuality, 133, 140, 146–165
    acceptance of body change
        and, 152–153
    aging and, 147–149
    communication and,
        148–150
    depression and, 158
    diminished libido,
        147–149
    doctors and, 162
    estrogen loss and, 147,
        155, 158–159
    hormone-replacement
        therapy and, 155–157
    hormones and, 147
    list of physical and sensual
        pleasures and, 153–154
    mastectomies and, 151
    painful intercourse, 156–
        160
    physical difficulties with,
        154–155
    position during
        intercourse, 160–161
    reticence of doctors to talk
        about, 148
    self-image and, 151
    sex therapists and, 162

Sexuality (*cont.*)
  sexual sensate exercises,
    154
  special concerns of single
    women, 162–165
  Viacream and, 161
  Viagra for women, 161
Sexual sensate exercises, 154
Single women, sexual con-
  cerns of, 162–165
Skin burns, 29
Sleep difficulties, 21, 45–47,
  70, 87
Soaps, 56
Social Security Disability
  (SSD), 216
Social workers, oncology, 261
Soy, hot flashes and, 74
Spirituality, 263–271
Stress, medical follow-up and,
  90–91
Stress-management
  programs, 255–256
Suicide, physician-assisted, 247
Supplemental Security In-
  come (SSI), 216
Support, 24–25, 44–45, 249–
  262
  advocacy, 260
  communicating about, 250
  emotions and
    psychological-support
    services, 44–45
  faith and, 251

friends in support groups,
    204
  online chat rooms or
    support groups,
    253–255
  previous experience and,
    251–252
  professionally-led groups,
    257–259
  psycho-educational or
    information groups,
    252–253
  psychotherapy, 46–47,
    260–262
  self-help groups, 256–257
  stress-management
    programs, 255–256
  value of, 249–250, 252
Surgery:
  axillary, 55–56, 64
  changes following, 52–56
  lumpectomy, 52, 64
  mastectomy, 52, 53, 64,
    151, 226, 240
  reconstruction, 53–55

Tamoxifen, 29, 36, 58, 103–
  116, 159
  vs. aromatase inhibitors, 113
  blood clots (thrombosis)
    and, 109–110
  breast cancer genes and,
    230–231

complications, 107–110

costs of, 111–112

dosage, 107

duration of treatment,
    104–105

estrogen-receptor negative
    breast cancer and, 105

estrogen-receptor positive
    breast cancer and, 105

fertility and, 170, 171

function of, 106

half-life of, 107

prevention of new breast
    cancers with, 105

resistance to use of, 116

screening for endometrial
    cancer and, 107–109

side effects, 110–111,
    115–116

Tamoxifen Breast Cancer
    Prevention Trial, 105

Tenderness, post-radiation,
    56–57

Terminology, 28

Testosterone, 147, 149, 157

Therapists, 136–137

Thrombosis, 109–110

Timetable of wellness, 39–43

Transvaginal ultrasound, 108–
    109

Treatment:
    alternative, 121
    chemotherapy, *See*
        Chemotherapy

complementary therapies,
    See Complementary
    therapies

finishing: the very first
    weeks, 15–38
    acute crisis, 21–22
    adaptation, 22–23
    apprehensions about
        health, 28–29
    emotions, 15–16, 19–
        21, 28, 30–32
    expectations of health,
        31
    feelings and type of
        treatment, 29–30
    giving yourself time,
        32–33
    new life, 26–27
    physical effects, 18–19,
        24, 27
    positive actions, 36–38
    rituals, 16–17, 36
    search for balance,
        33–35
    sense of abandonment,
        31
    support, 24–25
hormonal therapies,
    See Hormonal
    therapies
immediate aftermath of,
    39–50
    balance in daily life and
        routines, 40–41

Treatment (*cont.*)
    determining need for
      therapy, 46–47
    emotions and psycho-
      logical-support
      services, 44–45
    family and friends, 41–43
    normalcy of overpower-
      ing feelings, 47–48
    post-traumatic stress
      disorder (PTSD),
      45–46
    timetable of wellness,
      39–43
    tips for, 49–50
    radiation therapy, 17–18,
      28, 29, 56–58
    surgery, *See* Surgery
Two-week rule, 77, 89, 98

Ultrasound, breast, 91
Ultrasound, transvaginal,
    108–109

Vacations, 70–71, 140–141
Vaginal dryness, 156, 157,
    159–160
Viacream, 161
Viagra, 150, 161
Vitamin therapy, 120

Weight gain, 46–47, 58–60,
    110, 116
Weight loss, 46–47, 59–61
Wellness Community, 259
Work, *See* Professional issues
World Health Organization
    (WHO), 126

X rays, chest, 92–93

Y-Me, 259

Zorfass, Judith, 33

About The Author

HESTER HILL SCHNIPPER is Chief, Oncology Social Work, at Beth Israel Deaconess Medical Center in Boston, where she has worked since 1979. In 1993, after fourteen years of counseling breast cancer patients, she was diagnosed with the disease herself, an experience that has forged new bonds with the women with whom she works.

In 1999, Ms. Schnipper, who received her MSW degree from the Simmons College School of Social Work, was a recipient of the first Susan G. Komen Breast Cancer Foundation Survivor Professorship. She has taught and lectured widely in the field, is the author of numerous articles in professional journals, and has collaborated in two previous books for women newly diagnosed with breast cancer. She is married to Lowell E. Schnipper, MD, Professor of Medicine at the Harvard Medical School and Chief of the Division of Hematology/Oncology at Beth Israel Deaconess Medical Center.